WHAT PEOPLE ARE SAYING ABOUT

A Most Clarifying Battle

In this beautiful book that is both scholarly review and memoir, Dr. Vance describes the unique challenges and gifts of living with chronic illness. In an easy-to-read, clear style, Vance tells her story, interwoven with the stories of others, in such a way that we feel we too are riding the ups and downs of the chronic illness roller coaster. In exploring suffer⸱ loss, chronic illness as personal responsibility or ⸱ rtunity, and cancer as other or self, Vance ⸱ ⸱ representation of an experience t⸱ ⸱ hcare professionals, caregivers aı ⸱ ⸱ reading this book, and gain reso⸱ ⸱ journey. Looking at healing as a body-min⸱ ⸱ osition, Vance portrays the healing that can occur oı ⸱ ievels – emotional and spiritual, even when physical healing is not possible! With authenticity and grace, Landis Vance has shown us how to live out this view of wholeness, with its ups and downs, and how to achieve peace amidst chaos.
Christina Jackson, PhD, MSN, Professor of Nursing, Curriculum Committee Chair, Nursing Department, Eastern University

It is the rare voice that can give flight to the soul in adversity. Landis Vance is such a voice. Her heartfelt descriptions of coping with cancer, first as a chronic condition and now, as an overwhelming foe, opens our eyes to the fullness of living in the midst of life threatening hardship. *A Most Clarifying Battle: The Spirit and Cancer* must be read by everyone, ill and well.
Mark Langweiler, DC, DAAPM, Senior Lecturer, Anatomy, University of South Wales

This is both an informative and heart-wrenching book written by a woman who knows the cancer story from many perspectives. It is a series of articles, essays, and journal entries about her cancer experiences as a healthcare professional as well as her own journey. Her observations are acute, timely and very personal. Her story is shared without being maudlin, but totally honest, experience-in-the-moment. The overall message is that one needs to live life to the fullest, when possible, holed-up when not, and deeply connected to family, friends and one's personal gods... exercising as she has coined "spiritual muscle" to keep her consciousness present. Cancer is not the enemy; it is a part of her journey, a part of the struggles of her body, but never touching her eternal spirit.

Miriam Ratner, MSW, Psycho-oncologist, the Spectrum Center for Natural Medicine

A Most Clarifying Battle feeds the heart, mind, and spirit of people with cancer and their friends and families. Dr. Vance draws on her well-honed intellect to offer research results, ideas, and tools to help the reader approach the challenges of cancer. Drawing on experiences gleaned from her own multi-year battle with advanced cancer, she offers an inspiring personal story of courage, suffering, and perseverance. This book makes readers feel they have a wise companion who walks the cancer road by their side.

Joan Paddock Maxwell, MTS, Palliative Care Chaplain (ret.)

In recent years, I have tried to support several family members and friends as they battled the cancer roller coaster. I wanted to help, but felt powerless. I would have eagerly read Landis Vance's *A Most Clarifying Battle* had it been available. *A Most Clarifying Battle* gives powerful new insights into chronic illness and the interrelationship of spirituality, psychology, and medicine. By combining her practical theology and health

academic study, with hands-on work as a hospital chaplain, and a personal memoir of her own cancer journey – Dr. Vance offers insights into the physical, emotional, and spiritual challenges of living with cancer or chronic illness. This book would be useful to patients, physicians, medical personnel, and clergy as well as concerned family and friends.
Cathryn Seymour Dorsey, Care Provider

Landis Vance's *A Most Clarifying Battle* is an extraordinary exploration of what it means to journey through cancer... This inspiring book will be of immense inspiration not only for those who have a cancer diagnosis, but for their loved ones and friends as well. For anyone who doubts the importance of spirituality in health and illness, this book should be required reading.
Larry Dossey, MD, author, *One Mind: How Our Individual Mind Is Part of a Greater Consciousness and Why It Matters*

A Most Clarifying Battle

The Spirit and Cancer

A Most Clarifying Battle

The Spirit and Cancer

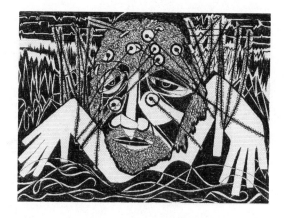

Landis M.F. Vance

BOOKS

Winchester, UK
Washington, USA

First published by O-Books, 2017
O-Books is an imprint of John Hunt Publishing Ltd., Laurel House, Station Approach,
Alresford, Hants, SO24 9JH, UK
office1@jhpbooks.net
www.johnhuntpublishing.com

For distributor details and how to order please visit the 'Ordering' section on our website.

Text copyright: Landis M.F. Vance 2016

ISBN: 978 1 78535 545 5
978 1 78535 546 2 (ebook)
Library of Congress Control Number: 2016945813

A CIP catalogue record for this book is available from the British Library.

Design: Stuart Davies

Printed and bound by CPI Group (UK) Ltd, Croydon, CR0 4YY, UK

We operate a distinctive and ethical publishing philosophy in all
areas of our business, from our global network of authors to
production and worldwide distribution.

CONTENTS

Other Works by the Author

(2015) "Issues in Spirituality Research in the Biomedical Context" in M.J. Langweiler and P.W. McCarthy (Eds.), *Methodologies for Effectively Assessing Complementary and Alternative Medicine (CAM): Research Tools and Techniques.* London: Singing Dragon, ISBN-13: 978-1848192515

(2007) *Spiritual Experiences of Chronic Illness When There is no Personal God.* Ann Arbor, ProQuest. UMI Number 3273547

(2003) "The Role of Culture in the Pain Experience." *The Pain Clinic: A Multidisciplinary Approach to Acute and Chronic Pain Management,* 5 (5), 10–23

Acknowledgements

Lyrics to *After This* by Elaine Dempsey, 1999. Copyright 2000 by Elaine Dempsey. Reprinted with permission.
Drawings by Csaba Osvath, 2003. Copyright 2003 by Csaba Osvath. Reprinted with permission.

Preface: Illness and Death are Spiritual Experiences

"Of the 12 or 13 suicides I've known, none of them had any interest in nature. In other words, they had no interest in what Rimbaud called 'the other,' the otherness, say, of nature." They could not make, [Jim] Harrison said, "that jump out of themselves."
Bissell, T., "The Last Lion," *Outside Magazine,* October 2011, p. 119

That "jump out of oneself," that connection to something "other," is Spirituality. Anyone who has a sense of connection to something "more" is spiritual. That connection can be to one's family, to the experience of listening to beautiful music, to the serenity of casting a fly rod on a beautiful river, or to the spiritual realm. And, if you have that sense of being connected, you are a spiritual 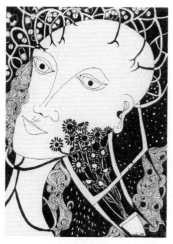 person. Even those who do not believe in a personal God are spiritual people, and this book, especially, is for you.

Here you will find various simple tools that you can use yourself to strengthen your own spiritual coping ability and to enhance your quality of life. And, you will hear my personal story as a person living with Stage 4 breast cancer: my struggles, worries, pain. I have included my story in the hope that you will be able to identify with parts of it, and that by reading it you will have a sense of how the experience and emotions of this disease change shape as time goes by. It is helpful for us to know that we are not alone. If you would like to stay in contact after reading this book, please visit my blog at www.spiritmountainwilds.com.

You will also find articles discussing research into the relationship between spirituality and illness. Sometimes it is nice to have science confirming our impressions (and it can help when we talk with our healthcare providers). Scientific research has found that when we are able to find meaning in the midst of chaos it acts as a critical force that can reduce suffering. This and similar findings are discussed in order to discover the many other aspects of the relationship between spirituality and health that lead to well-being and healing.

This book has been percolating for a few years and it is offered with great thanks to those of my fierce friends who believed in it and in me. To Jan Innes, thank you for starting the project off by refusing to allow the words to die. To Csaba Osvath, thank you for opening up your treasures of art to inspire me. To Maggie Logan and Nancy Rose, thank you for reading and discussing and editing and especially for helping me to not lose the beating heart of the work. And most especially to those who have been beside me over the years on this wild ride called cancer; you have not flinched but have carried me when I needed to be carried and treated me as a full person not a disease. And to BV for whom I fight to live.

So, welcome! I am glad you are here.

Landis M.F. Vance

Part I: Research into Illness, Suffering, and Spirituality

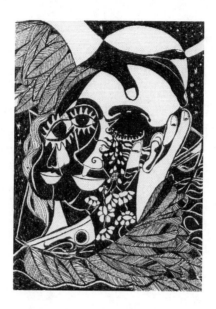

Chronic Illness, Suffering, and Society

In this book, I refer to cancer as a chronic disease. Most cancers are not chronic but, for those of us suffering with metastatic disease, the disease is chronic because there is no cure. Even in the few times when we are told that there is no evidence of disease, the physical toll of constant treatment, taken over years and not months, usually manifests in chronic side effects that impact function and quality of life.

There is an interior landscape of suffering that accompanies living with a chronic debilitating condition. It is unacknowledged but it affects relationships and undermines quality of life. Many of us are aware of it only to the extent that we may have a friend or family member who irritates us by not following through with social commitments or who always seems to be tired and not able to keep up.

Written accounts of living with a chronic illness all point to four overarching concerns which are discussed below:

Loss
Lack of reliability or consistency
Need for normalcy
Medical Team Fatigue

Loss in Chronic Illness

Some of the losses that come from living with a chronic illness include the loss of control over one's life and especially over one's own body, loss of educational or career opportunities, a loss of hopes and dreams as life will not turn out the way one had planned, and loss of self-respect as one moves from doing to just being. Frequently relationships are harmed and even broken. One patient said that he felt that he was "irrevocably and irretrievably damaged" (Gordon, 1997, p. 99).

The loss of control over one's life is particularly difficult. During the experience of chronic illness everything about life appears to be out of control. There are even limits to the power of your choices. Another patient wrote, "My choices were never final... My physical state was never constant" (Goldstein, 2000, pp. 95–96).

Reliability in Chronic Illness

This experience of loss and powerlessness is never over. There is never a time when you are done with a chronic illness. The way that one feels changes quickly and demands changes in treatment plans and in social plans. Both of these are difficult but the long-term effect of being considered to be "unreliable" in social terms can be devastating.

Frequently people who have chronic illness do not look sick and friends have no other way of judging their physical state or any way of understanding why plans have to be canceled or changed. Many times the sufferer is actually thought to be taking advantage of others rather than actually needing time to take care of her/himself. Some friends get disgusted and drop by the wayside.

Another thing that tends not to be recognized is that people have a need to contribute to the greater society, a need for what is known as "generativity." Living with a chronic illness makes this need both critical to one's sense of identity and well-being as well as an unavoidable reminder of one's infirmity. Generative activities, such as work or volunteer projects, frequently involve a requirement for being active at certain times and places. However, the nature of chronic illness makes this complicated, and often unmanageable, and may make it not only more difficult for someone with a chronic illness to contribute but also reduce the availability of opportunities to do so.

Chronic illness also goes through cycles of remission and recurrence which can be devastating. Most people who live with a chronic illness will tell you that relapses are made much worse by the fact that they follow temporary remissions when "we think, with the eternal optimism of well-being, that we have escaped the clutch of pain for good" (Duff, 1993, p. 16).

Normalcy in Chronic Illness

The need for normalcy is a need experienced by all people living with chronic illness, partly because dependability is a critical component in human experience and, more importantly, because illness and health are social constructions. Society expects that illness comes only in periods of limited duration (you either get well or you die). Although the person who is ill is certainly given permission to take the time necessary to heal, this permission begins to be denied the longer a patient is ill, and in time society begins to develop a sense that the person really isn't sick at all but is malingering.

This can often lead to the ill person trying to be normal, even

5

when feeling ill, lying when asked how he or she is doing by saying that she/he feels fine, and overestimating her or his strength or abilities. The person who is ill feels forced to create socially acceptable reasons for not living up to her or his potential.

If I had my way, I would tell anyone who inquired about my career ambitions that I remain in a less-than-satisfying job because of the security that it offers, and that I need the security to manage my life with bipolar disorder. I want an airtight excuse for what I perceive as my failure to make better use of my talents and education (Griesenbeck, 1997, p. 58).

Patients try to act normally in other ways by denying the reality of the illness or by erecting boundaries between the ill self and the normal self. Patients will offer differing accounts of how they are feeling depending on whether they are in a social or in a medical setting. Psychologically they may see themselves as two different people – the sick patient and the well individual – in an attempt to distance themselves from their illness.

People may be averse to using assistive devices, such as white canes or braces, because they call attention to their condition. This is one reason that cancer patients dread losing their hair during chemo; it marks them for all to see. Patients may also not want procedures that were once easily done in a clinic done instead by a home health nurse because it allows the illness to invade the sanctity of the home in a more tangible way (Goldstein, 2000).

Patients may want to hold on to items from their pre-illness life as talismans for the future. Melissa Goldstein (2000) writes about holding on to pairs of shoes that she would never be able to wear again because keeping them allowed her to hope that, one day, she would be able to dance. This speaks not only to coping but to the struggle to maintain one's identity.

Another aspect of the need for normalcy is the challenge to achieve a balance between dependency and independence. Friends and caregivers often do not understand how important it is for someone who is ill to be able to attend to little things. Caregivers may say with all good intention, "Here, let me. You shouldn't be doing that!" However, when they give too much it can, paradoxically, either increase the patient's felt need for independence and normalcy or may encourage the patient in a belief that he/she is incapable and therefore must be dependent in all things. Allan Macurdy, a person with muscular dystrophy, writes the following passage:

> Some have argued, therefore, that I should eliminate all sources of risk and protect myself at all costs, but that could happen only if I were willing to live apart from other people in some kind of bubble. I would not be able to teach, represent clients, see friends, have an intimate life with my wife, play with my nephews and godchildren, or hug my dog. In other words, all those things that give my life value, purpose, and meaning would be sacrificed in order to protect me from infections that might kill me. Who would want to have such a barren, empty life (Macurdy, 1997, pp. 14–15)?

Medical Fatigue in Chronic Illness

Every narrative I have come across includes what I call medical fatigue. This is where physicians, having tired of not being able to cure the patient, opt not to continue treating them. The suffering that results from this has an urgent threatening quality far surpassing the forms of suffering enumerated above. This area is so important that it is addressed more fully in the section More on Medical Fatigue below.

There is a lot that caregivers can do to lessen their suffering and the suffering of those for whom they care, but these issues must be acknowledged and caregivers need to become better informed, not just on the physical aspects of disease, but on the psychological and spiritual aspects. If you are interested in learning more, the patient narratives that have been referenced in this article can be found in the books listed below.

Duff, K. (1993) *The Alchemy of Illness*. New York: Bell Tower
    Goldstein, M.A. (2000) *Travels with the Wolf: A Story of Chronic Illness*. Columbus, OH: Ohio State University Press
    Young-Mason, J. (1997) *The Patient's Voice: Experiences of Illness*. Philadelphia: F.A. Davis Company

Communal Aspects of Illness

A major part of any consideration of illness is its communal nature. As those involved in cancer research are aware, disease infects an entire family, not just the person diagnosed. Family and friends suffer with their loved one.

Sometimes illness makes people uncomfortable. You can see this when a parent or friend holds onto a belief that if the patient would only try hard enough he/she will be healed, or the belief that there isn't anything really wrong. Other times the people that the patient thought would be there through anything just disappear from her/his life. Often they are overwhelmed by the burdens of care giving and of managing the day-to-day tasks that fall on them.

Families and friends are forced to renegotiate relationships in the face of chronic illness (Hunt, 2000). It is hard and lonely to be in this situation and those living with illness may feel that it is unfair that they are the ones who will have to reach out and attempt to bridge that space, like they don't have enough to do just being sick. The disease of the family is often unacknowledged and untreated.

However, if we are brave and acknowledge these problems and attempt to resolve them, this very renegotiation of relationships can result in a deepening of ties that become more meaningful and satisfying. Unexpectedly, a number of accounts noted that this renegotiation resulted not only in the caregiver's increased duties to the patient, but in the patient assuming care giving responsibilities for the caregiver, a mutuality of love, respect, and care springing from the experience of illness.

My husband and I have experienced this firsthand. The fact of my cancer had frightened him into avoiding the subject altogether. After a long time of my being honest with him about my needs and my fears for him, and encouraging him to speak about his own feelings, our relationship is much deeper, sweeter, and more satisfying and I have confidence that we have been able to develop the support that we will need towards the end of my life.

Mark Nepo expresses this quite well in a more poetic account of his experience with cancer:

> We are well because people didn't watch our suffering, but entered us and then felt love-suffering of their own. At times, this hurt them too much, which, in turn, forced us to nurture them, until, in bare, essential ways on certain days, we weren't sure who was ill and who was well – a solution that saved us all (Nepo, 1997, p. 137).

The communal nature of illness is not limited, however, to family and friends. It also includes the entire society. Illness and illness behaviors have societal definitions and a framework of rules. Illness also may have roots in the choices and values of a society that led to the development and promotion of environmental factors and that shape approaches to healthcare. For example, in the United States, along with the development of industry, came a concept of the body as machine. This in turn shaped which forms of healthcare would be acceptable and which would not. The allopathic system of medicine in Western culture is based on the idea of systems and mechanisms, not on the interrelationship between the soul and the world as is medicine in some other cultures.

This approach, for the most part, has also limited the focus of healthcare to considerations of the individual mechanism (the body of the patient) and not the ecology within which the mechanism (body) is placed. Thus, our approach to illness avoids considering the link between ozone depletion and melanoma, or other controllable environmental factors, and focuses on illness as a personal problem. The inability or disinterest of the society to reform the manner in which care is given and paid for reconfirms that illness in Western society is considered a personal problem (Kleinman, 1988).

Kat Duff believes that illness may be a cosmic form of societal scapegoating (Duff, 1993). She refers to the theory that society is out of balance (increasingly focused on material possessions and less in tune with natural phenomena); thus, balance must be achieved in a way that will humble society and allow it to take its rightful place in the universe.

"Such traditions," wrote Joseph Epes Brown, "affirm for those who listen, or indeed inevitably for those who do not, that where the sacred in the world and life is held as irrelevant illusion, where evasion of sacrifice in pursuit of some seeming 'good life' becomes a goal into itself, then... the ordering cycle of sacrifice will and must be accomplished by nature herself so that again there may be renewal in the world." As I understand it, the "ordering cycle" of nature most often manifests as natural disasters and disease epidemics, for "she" sleeps and stirs in the bowels of the earth, and our bodies. We have but one choice: to sacrifice or be sacrificed (Duff, 1993, p. 136).

Thus, according to Duff, those who become ill are functioning as scapegoats of society, the vehicles through which balance is being restored for all. She also refers to the phenomenon that many of those who have been ill frequently state their belief that their illness served some higher purpose, or that individuals may return from a period of illness with a passion to "set things right" as further evidence of this scapegoating function (Duff, 1993, pp. 114–115).

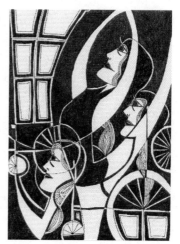

Duff, K. (1993) *The Alchemy of Illness*. New York: Bell Tower

Hunt, L.M. (2000) "Strategic Suffering: Illness Narratives as Social Empowerment among Mexican Cancer Patients." In C. Mattingly and L.C. Garro (Eds.), *Narrative and the Cultural Construction of Illness and Healing* (pp. 88–107). Berkeley: University of California Press

Kleinman, A. (1988) *The Illness Narratives: Suffering, Healing & the Human Condition*. New York: Basic Books

Nepo, M. (1997) "God, Self, and Medicine." In J. Young-Mason (Ed.), *The Patient's Voice* (pp. 132–143). Philadelphia: F.A. Davis Company

Illness as an Agent of Spiritual Transformation

Kat Duff, in her book *The Alchemy of Illness*, reminds us that "one of the central tenets of alchemical philosophy was that physical decay is the beginning of the 'Great Work'; *spiritual transformation*" (Duff, 1993, p. 79). [Italics mine for emphasis.] In 2007, while researching a study I was doing on the nature of spirituality in the chronically ill, I came across a number of patient narratives that described ways in which such individuals felt that they had been transformed through the process of living with their disease, and these transformations had a particularly spiritual feel to them. My own findings, which will follow below, support this.

Kat Duff, writing about her own illness experience, writes:

The alchemists insisted that two things must happen before the cure can be extracted from the disease. The problem must be kept in a closed container, and it must be reduced to its original state through a process of breakdown. The limitations and immobility of illness provide the closed container that enables this transformation, precisely because there is no way out (1993, p. 81).

Later in her text, she looks from alchemical philosophy to finding insight on the transformative power of illness in the form of initiation rituals:

When I woke from that dream I realized that my illness had come to serve the function of initiation, it was bequeathing me a mantle of power... These rites (initiation rites within traditional cultures) are not events so much as processes, transformations triggered by contact with the sacred, they are intended to prepare the individual for the powers, privileges, and responsibilities of the phase of life they are entering, by actually cultivating the strengths and awareness that will be needed (Duff, 1993, pp. 92–93).

In her account, Duff describes her encounter with sacred power with that which is so beyond human comprehension that it can only be approximated through the stories found in holy myth.

Mark Nepo, in his account of his bout with cancer, describes his spiritual experience:

Yet we have also been touched by a relentless, mysterious grace that has surfaced briefly to restore us. Repeatedly, it rises to save us or empower us – we can no longer make the distinction – and we find ourselves tied to a fathomless place where neither of us had dared to voyage. We call that reservoir God, although you may call it something else (Nepo,

1997, p. 134).

Melissa Goldstein expresses her encounter with the transcendent during her adjustment to life with lupus:

> The Light is the physical embodiment of all that I had sensed, and a great deal more, which I had vaguely intuited. The Light is my faith. I call upon it when the emotional or physical pain of my disease becomes unbearable. And it is through the image of my eagle that I join with the Light to find comfort... I looked to the sky with all that was in me. "Please be with me in my illness. Do not leave me alone in this terrible place." Then the ambient Light descended, washing in waves over me, and through me. I heard whispers, words of solace and healing. They were in a language beyond my conscious translation, but the sense of peace they brought me was total and complete. As the Light poured into me, filling me, I no longer spoke in words. For I was in the Light, part of the Light. I was Light. I did not need words to be heard (Goldstein, 2000, pp. 29–30).

Although not all of the narratives I read were able to express the spirituality of their illness as clearly, they all referred to it being a time where they were able to find meaning in their suffering and to come to know themselves in a way that was deeper and more complete than before. An account of a patient, who had a near-death experience during surgery, stated that if he had the choice he would rather not have gone through the experience at all. Nevertheless, at the end of his story he says:

> For a while I was afraid I would lose something I had nearly died to obtain and might never have a chance to find again... I thought that if I didn't adhere strictly to the insights and intuitions released during the near-death experience, I would

lose everything I'd gained from it, and all I'd have left in the end would be the pain and the loss. The whole struggle, I thought, would have been in vain. Now I think that the jewel is not so easily discarded (Gordon, 1997, p. 101).

In another passage, he adds:

In the end, I'm not sure what it all means or if it means anything really. One thing I know is that coming that close to death makes you aware of choices you didn't know you had before. And they are not small choices; they are all the choices there are (Gordon, 1997, p. 103).

In the narratives that I read it appeared that the way these individuals were able to arrive at such knowledge and experience was through an active engagement with their illnesses, by not being passive in their suffering. Donna Griesenbeck writes of her experience of bipolar disease:

I can, however, identify a progression from a strict church-bound religiosity toward a broader spirituality, a progression that parallels my personal development over the same time… Whatever the underlying biophysical reality, I am convinced that the suppression of my creative and spiritual self also contributed to my experiences of psychosis. By integrating the interpretation of my psychotic experiences into my everyday life, I am able to reclaim neglected aspects of my authentic self. As I more consciously develop my creativity, I believe that I lessen the likelihood and the severity of another episode.

The experiences I have described illustrate how the challenge of altering my self-concept to integrate my experiences with mental illness led to significant personal growth (Griesenbeck, 1997, p. 58).

In my own study, the patient who disagreed that her experience had any spiritual elements, stating that God had nothing to do with her experience of illness and that she did not expect any great change, did express to me that she had been subtly transformed. She said that while she did not experience anything that she would call "spiritual," she did see a change in her life since her diagnosis: she was living more authentically and more respectfully, acknowledging her own desires. In this she has experienced a heightened connection to her own self. "Yes, that's what I want to be. I just want to be, I guess, true to myself. I just don't want to play games with me anymore. I know my qualities and I know my faults" (Vance, 2007, pp. 171–172).

Another person who participated in my research project was dealing with life as an alcoholic. He said to me, "You know, I would like to think too that great cosmic things are guiding me. It's always fun to be grandiose… especially if you want a drink… but then I found if I had a big dinner, or just a milkshake, or something, that the craving was much less, which is almost… well, in a way it's deflating because you think, 'Oh no! This is a deep profound spiritual need. A milkshake isn't going to do anything.' Well, actually a milkshake is the cure at that particular moment. Something as routine and banal as that will save my life" (Vance, 2007, p. 172). This too is indicative of a spiritual experience, finding the potential for the sacred in the everyday. In his case, his transformation was hard won over decades and brought him to a place of living authentically, a place of peace.

My own experiences living with a series of significant illnesses, most recently metastatic cancer, have been the catalyst for positive change, for making choices I had not been brave enough to make in the past, all of which has led me to joy and peace as well. My illness is what keeps me on that path. It is the voice that speaks loudly to me of the need to take care of myself, and that gives others an opportunity to show that I am loved. Illness can indeed be a powerful force for positive life enhancing change and can provide us with more intimate knowledge of the ways in which we are connected to ourselves, each other, the world around us, and even to God but it is something that demands that we engage with it.

It is a modern day retelling of the story of Jacob wrestling with the angel and refusing to let the angel go until he had received his blessing. When the battle was over, Jacob was transformed forever, he had a new identity (Israel) and he walked with a limp but he also had received a blessing that would never be taken from him (Genesis 32:22–32).

Duff, K. (1993) *The Alchemy of Illness*. New York: Bell Tower

Goldstein, M.A. (2000) *Travels with the Wolf: A Story of Chronic Illness*. Columbus, OH: Ohio State University Press

Gordon, D. (1997) "Reconceptions." In J. Young-Mason (Ed.), *The Patient's Voice: Experiences of Illness* (pp. 75–105). Philadelphia: F.A. Davis Company

Griesenbeck, D. (1997) "Psychosis: Art, Life, or Illness?" In J. Young-Mason (Ed.), *The Patient's Voice: Experiences of Illness* (pp. 55–61). Philadelphia: F.A. Davis Company

Nepo, M. (1997) "God, Self, and Medicine." In J. Young-Mason (Ed.), *The Patient's Voice* (pp. 132–143). Philadelphia: F.A. Davis Company

Vance, L.M.F. (2007) *Spiritual Experiences of Chronic Illness when There is No Personal God*. Ann Arbor, MI: ProQuest

More on Medical Fatigue

Medical Fatigue is a phenomenon that has only recently begun to be discussed. It is a great source of spiritual suffering that is familiar to most, if not all, individuals coping with a chronic illness. If you are suffering from a chronic illness that is debilitating, you will have experienced this phenomenon. If you are caring for someone you may have experienced it as well from the other side in your own thoughts, the kind that usually start,

"Why can't s/he just..."

Medical Fatigue and the Diagnosis

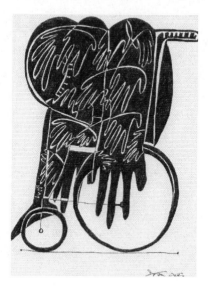

Many chronic illnesses are difficult to diagnose; the average time to diagnose lupus, for example, is three years (Goldstein, 2000). In the time preceding diagnosis, the patient is often told (especially women patients) that there is nothing wrong with him or her, or that it is all in her or his mind. This lack of being believed by physicians is a major contributor to patients' spiritual suffering, for it causes them to begin to doubt their own perceptions in the midst of their physical suffering, and it affects their sense of self-worth, acceptability, and lovability. Further, not being believed diminishes their personhood and dignity, increases a sense of hopelessness and can actually increase physical pain and suffering (Brady et al., 1999; Clark, 2000).

Melissa Goldstein (2000, p. 45) expresses the frustration of this experience:

I've been through this so many times before. Doctors are faced with symptoms they cannot explain. So they paste on a psychosomatic label, because they don't know what else to say. A few weeks or months later, the doctors find out what is really causing my medical problems. But in the meantime, I'm bounced to the psychiatrists, who declare that I'm perfectly healthy emotionally, and that my problems are not psychiatric. I then get tossed back to the medical people. I'm not a ping pong ball; *I'm a human being. I'm tired of playing this game, and I won't do it anymore.* [Italics added for emphasis.]

Many who have written on this topic believe that physicians respond this way when they don't know what is wrong but cannot allow themselves to admit it; thus, their response transforms their own fear of professional inadequacy into questions of whether or not the patient is giving an adequate description of a real physical situation (Goldstein, 2000; Mairs as cited in Duff, 2000).

The value of a diagnosis in naming the experience of a patient is incalculable. It means that there really is something wrong; the patient now has credibility with the medical establishment. After months or years of not being believed, the diagnosis has the power to energize the physician into purposeful action.

Naming has always had mystical power in human experience and, just as it was once thought that if you named something you had control over it, patients (and perhaps physicians) feel that if the disease has a name, the doctors will be able to control it. But, with chronic illness, patient experiences suggest that this enthusiasm is short-lived as the disease does not often follow its expected course.

Medical Fatigue and Spiritual Suffering

As mentioned above, in dealing with patients who suffer from chronic illness many physicians experience medical fatigue, or compassion fatigue, because the disease is not curable but yet it demands treatment. Many patient accounts refer to this as a time when the physician appears to "turn" on the patient or to discharge her or him for no apparent reason. Other times a physician may be threatened when the patient asks for opinions from other physicians. One patient describes the battle that ensued between services at a local hospital because one service questioned the treatment being provided by the other; this battle ended up with the patient being "fired" by the first service (Goldstein, 2000).

Patients transfer onto their physicians their hopes for and beliefs in a future with less physical suffering. Fear, of not only the disease but also inadequate treatment, adds another layer of meaning and emotion for patients who have given their trust to a physician; there is a sense of comfort and security that patients project onto their doctors that makes being discharged under these circumstances a devastating form of betrayal. Leaving a doctor, care team, or hospital that has been the focus of one's healing is also anxiety producing for many patients, and further compounds the spiritual and emotional pain.

Biomedical Culture Increases Spiritual Suffering

When medical or physician fatigue enters the patient relationship it is highly toxic, but there is much about the medical culture in general that contributes to patients' spiritual suffering. Medical personnel frequently refer to patients by the names of their conditions or procedures, when talking among themselves, rather than by the patients' personal names. While in the patient's room, physicians often ignore the patient and talk instead to others, or among themselves, about the patient's condition. This is even more likely if the patient is elderly, a child, does not speak English, or is disabled in some way. Allan Macurdy gives an example of this:

There I was in this intensive care unit, fevered, my lungs full of secretions, and unable to get enough air. Such circumstances are frightening enough by themselves. In the midst of all that activity, my anxiety was heightened by the fact that no one was listening to me; no one seemed to be aware that I existed beyond the data in my chart. But more terrifying still was the iron lung, and the procedure necessary to being placed inside... None of the residents seemed to notice, however. At a time when the right words could have allayed my fear... I met words that trivialized and excluded. The residents chattered on among themselves with great enthusiasm... But direct interaction with me consisted of awkward perfunctory monologues, delivered with impatience and never followed by listening (Macurdy, 1997, p. 11).

When physicians need to give bad news, they are frequently reported as standing close to the door, out of reach of the patient. They may become extremely interested in finding something in the patient's chart so as to avoid eye contact. Patients are told that they have "failed" the treatment plan, not that the treatment prescribed has failed them. This is interpreted as meaning that it is somehow the patient's fault that there was no improvement. Although these signs may be subtle, they are nonetheless powerful in adding to the patient's spiritual burden.

I am glad to say, however, that many medical schools have become aware of these issues and are attempting to train the new generation of physicians in the ways of more positive doctor-patient interactions. However, the specific issue of how to protect physicians from medical fatigue related to treating patients with chronic illnesses has yet to be addressed to my knowledge. As our population ages, chronic illness will become the predominant consumer of healthcare dollars and physician resources. The impact of medical fatigue on the provision of patient care must be addressed by medical school and professional associations.

Duff, K. (1993) *The Alchemy of Illness*. New York: Bell Tower
Goldstein, M.A. (2000) *Travels with the Wolf: A Story of Chronic Illness*. Columbus, OH: Ohio State University Press
Macurdy, A. (1997) "Mastery of Life." In J. Young-Mason (Ed.), *The Patient's Voice: Experiences of Illness* (pp. 9–17). Philadelphia: F.A. Davis Company

Spiritual Well-being in Coping with Illness

In 2002 Pam McGrath, in an article in *Supportive Care in Cancer*, explored the ways in which the crisis of having a serious illness will precipitate a time of disorientation. In this article she points out that the threatening nature of the illness, in conjunction with the demands of aggressive and invasive treatment, creates a disconnection or break with the normal or expected. These losses are experienced in the following categories:

Physical: hair loss, infertility, early menopause, and intense physical pain or duress.

Identity: loss of the patient's identity, loss of work and education, financial loss, and ultimately the loss of a sense of self.

Relational: stress in relationships with family and friends and, not uncommonly, the loss of these relationships.

Existential: loss of naïveté and cosmic loneliness.

These losses then lead one to begin to question the meaning of life. Although patients experience this in varying degrees of intensity, when it is experienced as acutely painful, it becomes spiritual pain (McGrath, P., 2002).

Dame Cicely Saunders, the founder of the Hospice movement, in her conceptualization of "total pain" includes four components:

Physical: degeneration, assaults to the integrity of the body.

Psychological: assaults to hope and dignity.

Social: isolation, loss of personhood.

Spiritual: loss of meaning (Clark, D., 2000, July/August).

Much research indicates that any one of these components can have an impact on the others. Just as physical pain can cause psychological pain, social, psychological, and spiritual pain can heighten the physical perception of pain. This affects not only the use of pain management drugs, but also the response to treatment experienced by the patient, and the degree to which the patient follows the prescribed treatment regimens.

An example of this dynamic can be taken from my experiences while a chaplain at a large research hospital. A 34-year-old Hispanic patient in the bone marrow transplant unit had successfully undergone a transplant, but she did not get better, in fact she got worse. The doctors tried everything and had no idea why she wasn't getting better.

About six weeks after the transplant, the patient made a passing comment to one of the nurses that she (the patient) was cursed. The nurse, rather than trying to distract the patient and make her feel better, asked her what she meant. When the patient began to talk, a story came out that the patient had tried healing during a Santeria service prior to entering the hospital for the procedure. At the conclusion of the ritual, the Santeria priest had demanded a large sum of money from her which she could not pay. At that moment the Santeria priest then cursed her and said that she would then pay either with her life or the life of her, then unborn, child.

For this patient, the failure to benefit from the treatment was her way of protecting the life of her child. The doctors had known nothing of this and were horrified. It would require serious long-term spiritual care if the patient was to be freed from the curse and to benefit from the transplant.

The reverse of this is also true: patients that are spiritually healthy have higher quality of life regardless of their life-condition than do those who are not. These patients have a greater sense that their life makes sense and a greater sense of peace. In 1999 a study done by Marianne Brady and others, and published in the *Journal of Psycho-Oncology* (vol. 8, pp. 417–428), found that spiritual well-being remained an important predictor of one's quality of life even when other factors such as one's physical state, emotional state, and social support or family well-being were considered. Of those who reported high levels of fatigue in this study, but also claimed that their life had meaning and said that they were at peace, 66% reported that they were still able to enjoy their lives very much.

On the other hand, only 11% of those who reported similar high levels of fatigue could say the same if they reported that their life had little meaning or peace.

These studies are only a few of those that have been done that indicate that spiritual well-being is an important ingredient in the overall experience of serious disease. It may be that the same results will hold for those experiencing any type of crisis. Spiritual well-being does matter in life.

Brady, M.J.; Peterman, A.H.; Fitchett, G.; Mo, M.; Cella, D. (1999) "A case for including spirituality in quality of life measurement in oncology." *Psycho-Oncology*, 8, 417–428

Clark, D. (2000, July/August) "Total pain: The work of Cicely Saunders and the hospice movement." *APS Bulletin*, 10(4). Retrieved May 20, 2006, from American Pain Society Web site: http://www.ampainsoc.org/pub/bulletin/ju00/hist1.htm

McGrath, P. (2002) "Creating a language for 'spiritual pain' through research: a beginning." *Supportive Care in Cancer*, 10, 637–646

Spiritual Tools: Building Strong Spiritual Muscle Helps Minimize Pain and Suffering

The study by Marianne J. Brady, that we have discussed before, indicates from a scientific perspective that there is a direct correlation between spiritual well-being and patients who report less fatigue and less pain even when the physical characteristics of their disease indicate significant physical impairment (Brady, et al., 1999). So how can we develop spiritual well-being if we are not finding spiritual advisers up to the task of helping us?

Fortunately for us, there is a long history of spiritual exercises being used by various groups to develop spiritual muscle. Whether it be Christian monastics or Zen monks, there is a body of work that can lead us to time tested activities that will produce results for our spirit the same way that going to the gym produces results for our bodies. But fair warning, just as it is easy to avoid going to the gym by piling up a raft of reasons why you are too busy, it is even easier to avoid these spiritual exercises because they can be uncomfortable and on some days you just aren't feeling it.

It takes a certain amount of bravery to take on becoming spiritually strong because during the course of these exercises we meet ourselves in our least flattering light. The first thing I want to do when this happens is to throw the unflattering me under the carpet and pretend it isn't even in the room, but oh so slowly I come to understand what C.G. Jung calls the "shadow" part of me. And just as slowly the shadow shows me what I need to acknowledge about myself and what I need to work on in order to get spiritually stronger.

So, what follows are simple exercises drawn from those who have gone before us. These exercises can be woven into any part of your day to help you become a stronger and more resilient person when faced with suffering in any of its forms.

Joy

We don't tend to think of the experience of joy as a spiritual tool. However, mystics write about being filled with joy. Holy writings often display humor and talk about the spiritual life as being filled with joy. The word ecstatic originally meant filled with the spirit and we understand it as being joyful.

So here is a tool that doesn't take time or a lot of effort. Think about what makes you happy, what fills you with a deep joy, and then make time in each day to focus on that. Holding a baby, being transported by beautiful music, there are many ways that we experience joy.

Keep a listing in your journal about where you find joy each day. Attune yourself to joy in your life. These moments are windows into the spirit world and provide peace.

Now joy and laughter are not the same thing, but they often go together. From a physiological perspective laughter promotes relaxation. One breathes more deeply when one laughs. Studies have shown that immune function is improved during laughter. Laughter helps to put things into proper perspective.

When I was first diagnosed with cancer I was scared to death, literally shaking with fear. My doctor gave me a packet of materials to take home and digest while waiting for my surgery date, and in this packet was a little book called *Cancer Has Its Privileges* (Clifford, C. and Lindstrom, J., 2002, New York: Perigee). It was a book about the funny side of having cancer – and yes, there really is a funny side. I remember sitting in the middle of my bed and crying I was laughing so hard. It took the sting out of the diagnosis. It was a moment of grace in a difficult period.

Labyrinths

Walking a labyrinth has long been a practice that results in connection to the sacred, in calmness and serenity, and increased clarity of focus. The explosion in interest and in the actual construction of labyrinths in the United States is due in large part to work that the Rev. Lauren Artress of Grace Cathedral, San Francisco has done to bring the practice to public attention, both through her book, *Walking a Sacred Path: Rediscovering the Labyrinth as a Spiritual Practice* (1996, New York: Riverhead Books), and information made available on the Cathedral's Web site. Since that time many hospitals and hospices have begun to include labyrinths on their grounds, acknowledging the particular benefits that this practice offers to those in physical or spiritual distress.

Using a labyrinth does not take any special gifts, all it takes is your intention. Many locations offer the use of their labyrinths to the public free of charge. You can find the location of the nearest labyrinth near you through the World-Wide Labyrinth Locator or you can purchase a finger labyrinth for your personal use. While

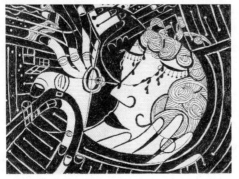 I was doing hospital chaplaincy I had a 16" finger labyrinth made from Corian that I used with patients who were not able to walk but who could benefit from the practice. The Corian was used because it was easy to maintain and could be disinfected between uses.

A labyrinth is basically a path that you follow from an entry point into the center of a design. Usually, once the center has been reached, the person walking rests there for awhile before retracing her/his steps back out again. The same thing is done with a finger labyrinth, only instead of walking one uses one's finger to trace the path.

You cannot get lost in a labyrinth. Unlike its cousin, the maze, which was designed to trick and fool people, labyrinths were designed so that you would find your way and not get lost. Often people are afraid of "doing it wrong" or of getting lost, but that will not and cannot happen here.

To start a labyrinth walk, come to the labyrinth with a question or an intention (need for calmness, need for answer, need to feel more connected). Pause at the beginning of the path to consciously acknowledge your intention and then begin slowly and reflectively to follow the path laid out before you. Do not seek to marshal your thoughts but just let them float freely as you notice what they are. Remember to let go; you cannot get lost so don't worry about how to get from here to there, just breathe and walk.

When you get to the center of the labyrinth take some time to reflect on your walk and the thoughts that came to you. Often people may sit or even lie down in the center for awhile. Then, when you feel that you are ready to return, acknowledge your gratitude for the experience and then return to the entrance, walking slowly reflecting on what you have gained.

Sometimes the experience feels like you haven't gained anything but, perhaps, some quiet time to yourself. That is OK. That is what you need. Other times you will have other experiences that may lead to insight on particularly vexing problems, or just a stronger sense of well-being. Sometimes these experiences may raise painful issues that need to be addressed rather than avoided. Whatever you experience here is what you are meant to experience in this particular time.

To work with a finger labyrinth is much the same. There are many different finger labyrinths available. Some are small and "walked" with a pointer and some are large with a groove in which you place your finger and follow to the center. There are some that are downloaded from the Internet and printed on paper, and others made from various types of wood or stone. If you would like to work with a finger labyrinth I recommend getting a larger one, 16" or so, in the "Chartres" pattern that has a groove that your finger feels comfortable in. You can find many vendors on the Internet.

Part of the function of the labyrinth is to keep the cognitive functioning of one's brain busy so that the normal self-criticism of which we all are guilty is focused on the activity and not on the part of the brain open to inspiration. Inspiration is more likely to come to you under these conditions. Because of this neurological fact, when I use finger labyrinths with clients I require that they use the ring finger of their non-dominant hand (i.e. the left hand if they are right-handed) and that they "walk" the labyrinth with their eyes closed.

This can be a very disorienting experience. People who are high achievers are always worried about not doing things correctly or not excelling. A psychologist that I worked with hated the exercise because she, as a high achiever, was so afraid of not doing it correctly, especially in front of another person. I do not think it is an overstatement to say that she hated this exercise with a passion because inevitably her movements would be herky-jerky and her hand would bounce off the board.

Nevertheless we kept at it until one day while she had her eyes closed she let go and felt a grand sweeping motion of her hand that she later said felt like flying. That was the turning point for her in her quest to learn to let go of her need to control everything about her life. So don't give up if this is your experience as well; good things will come out of it.

Lectio Divina: Meditation on a text

There is a form of guided meditation called Lectio Divina, or Holy Reading, that has been used for centuries. It is a series of repetitive reading of the same sacred text with periods of silence in between for contemplation and inspiration. This can be done both in group settings and when one is meditating alone. While it is often found as a spiritual discipline among Christians, in fact, this tool can be used with any text that the person meditating finds to be meaningful.

First choose a text that you would like to use as the basis of your meditation. There are no limits on the type of text that you can use, but make sure that it is not too long. A paragraph at the most will be easier to work with than a longer text.

Center yourself and calm your thinking. This can be done by taking a few minutes and focusing solely on your breathing, counting the seconds to breathe in, how long you hold your breath, and how long it takes you to breathe out each time.

If you are a person of prayer, use this time to pray being thankful for this time and offering yourself up to the wisdom that is to be revealed to you.

Read the text.

Now that you have read it once, and are familiar with it, read it again paying particular attention to what jumps out at you this time.

Take a few moments to reflect on what you have read (or heard if in a group) and note it in your mind.

Read the text again and take note of what jumps out at you this time. Is it the same or is it different, a different word or phrase?

Take a few minutes to reflect on this. How do these words/phrases relate to your life? How do you feel right now? What might this mean?

Read the text one last time slowly. What strikes you now?

Take a moment to center yourself again and then reflect on this experience. Sit with this for 2–5 minutes. If you would like, use this time to journal about what you have discovered.

When you have completed your journaling end the session by centering yourself again, acknowledging your gratitude for the inspiration or experience and, if it is appropriate, set an intention based upon what you have discovered within yourself.

Mandalas

Mandalas are nearly as old as time and can be found in many cultures. The word "mandala" means: whole world, healing circle, or center of the Universe in which a fully awakened being abides. They are full of sacred meaning. I have always viewed mandalas as being maps of the spirit.

There are many books and Web sites devoted to mandalas today. Some are coloring books where the act of coloring in the patterns can be an aid to meditation, but I prefer using the model of mandalas found in Tibetan Buddhism. In Tibetan Buddhism mandalas are designed using a specific code. They are meant to represent the universe as seen from looking down on the center of a temple.

The center of the mandala holds a representation of the Buddha, their most holy figure, surrounded by lines representing the outline of the temple structure. In circles which radiate from the center are usually symbolic representations of ordinary life and symbols of protection with the outer boundary representing a protective force.

The most meaningful mandala is the one that you develop on your own as an aid to your self-understanding and healing. You do not need to be an artist to do this. You can use a pattern of symbols OR you can use my trick and make a collage from images and text found in magazines and newspapers. If you choose to make a collage follow these instructions using the cutouts rather than drawings.

Take a piece of paper and draw a round circle.

Beginning at the center draw something which has meaning for you and represents the most important thing in your life.

Next draw a symbol of a quality that you have within you that protects this most important source of meaning.

Then in as many concentric circles as you would like, draw symbols for your life and symbols of what threatens you and what protects you, always placing what protects you closer to the center and what threatens you closer to the outside ring.

Use the outer circle to represent the absolute boundary of the universe as you know it.

Keep your mandala with you and study it from time to time. It will give you insight into your values, sense of meaning, and sense of place within the universal. Do not be surprised if the images that have meaning for you change periodically. When you feel that your interior landscape has changed, it might be helpful to do this exercise again.

The most common form of spiritual suffering is a lack of

authenticity. This exercise helps you to get in touch with what really is the most important to you and then gives you a symbolic visual reminder that you can keep with you on your spiritual journey.

One of my favorite Web sites shows a teacher who uses this type of exercise with her students. Using this link http://www2.lhric.org/pocantico/tibet/mandalas.htm will access the site and you will be able to see what the students came up with. Some are funny and some are sad, but they are all interesting windows into each child's particular world.

Part II: My Personal Experiences of Illness

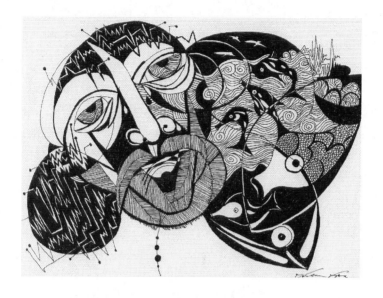

Save Me from the Pink Ribbons

What follows are various essays written at various times during the past seven years. They look at the issues surrounding living with metastatic breast cancer through the eye of a participant observer. These are the issues of that world as they are experienced with all of the paradoxes and dark humor that come into view.

The experience of having cancer changes over time; what concerned me when I was first diagnosed is no longer an issue seven plus years later on. When you are first diagnosed the experience of going in for CT scans is highly stressful. We even have a term for it: scanxiety. After over 30 scans, I no longer get anxious; it is just another friggin' doctor's appointment (and yes, your impatience at having to have another medical appointment does grow over time). So these essays were written at specific times and reflect my issues at the time they were written, not the current time. Cancer is truly a paradoxical experience and issues spool out in front and then double back to hit you from behind. My hope is that this book encourages others living with metastatic cancer to know they are not alone, however long they may have been on this journey, and to continue to live their lives to the fullest.

I Hate Pink Ribbons

I've been living with cancer for a long time and one thing I can categorically state is I hate pink ribbons! I hate the "rah rah beat cancer" culture that has been spawned by well-meaning individuals garnering support for cancer research. It invades my life and somehow I feel there must be a big L on my forehead for not being able to get into the spirit of things.

Don't get me wrong, I have done my share of pink ribbon events but I increasingly experience the ribbons as accusing me of moral weakness for not beating the cancer. A large number of invisible women are living with metastatic cancer. We are invisible because who wants to hear in this culture that we didn't beat the cancer. We also have mixed feelings about people knowing we still have this disease because who needs to have people look at you with sympathetic eyes that really mean "We are so sorry that you are going to die." I mean who needs that? The truth is that now it is possible to live with cancer for a long time.

Life with cancer can be good. I mean really good. It is full of all sorts of funny and odd moments. It is full of a new realization of what life can be and, if you are lucky and can be honest with your friends and partners, it can be a time of deep intimacy. It is also full of moments of mind-numbing fear about the future, but in time I have come to an accommodation with this part of the experience.

I call my tumors my roaches. They are like the roaches I used to have in my apartment: one day you treat for them and they disappear, a little later someone else treats for them and they skitter on back only to skitter away again. It's like that. For now, my roaches and I are just hanging out. They are kind of quiet and life is very good.

"Am I My Cancer?" and Other Heresies

In the pink ribbon world, we chant, "Rah, rah, beat cancer!" So cancer must be the enemy, some invader that has attacked us, right? We must believe this since the alternative that cancer might not be the enemy or that it might have come from our own selves, if true, would rock our world!

My friend, the scientist, and I had a heated exchange of views one day when I disagreed with this cancer framework by saying that I thought that my cancer is just that, my cancer. It is my cells that for some unknown reason have gone rogue. Many e-mails flew back and forth. His anxiety and perplexity rose as I, also a trained behavioral scientist, challenged this medical shibboleth.

When I went through treatment the first time I saw cancer as Other, "not me." But, I viewed it as a benevolent other, sort of like a medical angel that had been sent to teach me some life lesson. That is all well and good when you have an expectation that treatment, however horrific, will be successful and that once you have learned your lesson the cancer will go away and never visit again. There are many cancer books and visualization tapes that promote this idea. So I was very intent on being grateful to my cancer.

However, having metastatic disease really pulls the rug out from under you. There is all sorts of room for self-recrimination: was I not grateful enough, did I not learn the lesson I was to learn, and on and on. This is made even worse when I learned that the treatment that almost killed me did not, in fact, kill the cancer and that I am dealing with original cancer seeds.

The dichotomy between cancer as Other and one's Self can be the source of tremendous psychological and spiritual distress for those of us living with this disease. But, the tensions dissolve if I can turn this around and say that these cancer cells are part of me (but not all of me). A doctor friend of mine keeps reminding me that it is not the cells present in one's body but what one's body does with those cells that should be of concern.

Those of us who have been exposed to psychology understand the concept of the psyche's Shadow. I have come to believe that my cancer cells are the physical equivalent of the Shadow. As with a number of women, my physical self has been the dumping ground for all of those things about myself that I reject. (I'm too fat. I'm not pretty. I'm too clumsy, etc.) I was brought up in an evangelical Protestant home and was set up from birth to think of the world as a duality between good and evil as expressed by spirit and physical world. I reject all of that thinking now, but that training is deep in my unconscious.

I have learned from my work as a behavioral scientist that the Shadow is fertile ground for spiritual as well as psychological growth, and that when we are open to our Shadow selves the great mystery of life speaks to us with great power. I now believe that my cancer has been a metaphor for all that was diseased in my life. I am not surprised that my cancer is expressed as breast cancer because, as with most women, I have had people metaphorically attached to my tits my entire life. So, my nurturing self was worn-out and some of those nurturing relationships were toxic, thus my breasts became diseased.

After a great deal of thought, I have also come to the realization that the cancer might have arisen from my need to be protected and my body's attempt to do just that. I can finally say that the cancer has given me permission to put myself first and care for myself for the first time in my life. It has made me appreciate just how sweet and precious life is and how I had spent my former life pursuing values that mean nothing in the final analysis. Because of my disease I am now forced to slow down, live thoughtfully and intentionally, and to let those I love know that I love them. Because of the cancer, my relationships are now healthy and life-giving. And because my cancer will be around for the rest of my life, I will always have that stern but loving force sitting behind me ready to tap me on the shoulder and keep me on the road to wholeness if not cure.

Cancer and Loving Oneself

Earlier this year I underwent two massive surgeries where my cancer tumors were excised from my lungs. Being rid of the tumors, I was going to be back on top of my game. Or, that is what I thought, that I would go back to being the way I was before my cancer came back. So, when I get tired or when I can't do what I want to do during the day I get angry with myself and wonder what in the world is wrong with me. Of course the thought never enters my head that I have cancer. I don't know how to interpret this. Is it a positive thing that I continue to look so far past my disease that it fades away in my consciousness? Or, is it a negative thing, that I am so out of touch with my body that I lose track of its exact state and needs?

The past few days have been frustrating. I was doing well and then the norovirus swept our little valley and I contracted it. It only lasted about a week but since then I have had a hard time bouncing back. Tonight while I was once again wondering what was wrong with me, the realization finally came shimmering into my consciousness that I have been in active treatment for my cancer for over four years now. Four years of taking very strong medicine that progressively takes its toll on my body.

My red cell counts are falling. They have been since last September. No matter what I do I cannot get them back into normal range. I know this because every time I have chemo (really biologics and hormone treatments) I get a copy of my blood test and it shows my red cells are low, and my hematocrit, and my monocytes, etc. I suppose that is why I don't feel good. I don't have enough of whatever these are to do whatever it is they do. I guess it makes me feel better to have something "scientific" I can point to to say I really don't feel well. Why is it that the fact that I don't feel well is not sufficient? Why do I have to have corroboration from some impartial source? That is sad. That makes me very sad to know this about myself.

I have always found it very hard to love myself when I am ill, to allow myself to sleep in a soft bed and to coddle myself, to spoil myself. Instead I go around feeling anxious and vaguely guilty and keep trying to do all of the things that I "should" be doing and, obviously, failing. I guess it is that Puritan ethic and a childhood of only being loved for what I did rather than for who I was.

This cancer continues to be my teacher. Most of the lessons are painful but they all seem to be calling me to an intrinsic fullness of life: not the fullness of life that others can see, but an interior sense of well-being and peace, of acceptance and self-love that has always eluded me. Maybe I will finally get it before the end, I hope so. I think that is the basic lesson of life, that you have to start by loving and accepting yourself before you can love and accept others.

Wish me luck!

Finding a Rabbit in a Hat: Miracles in Cancer Treatment

So, dear reader, life with cancer is a life full of questions for which there are no sure answers. I am frequently in a quandary of whether or not to go back on chemo. While this may seem like there should be a simple answer, for me chemo is highly problematic. I have been fighting this disease off and on for 6 years. Every time that I have had chemo I have ended up in the hospital an infinitesimally small sliver away from death. It may be true that I will die from this disease but I prefer to die from the disease not from the treatment for the disease!

My friends and family were concerned that I was giving up

when I decided to not have more chemo. They began to treat me carefully as though I had begun the final journey. But I had not given up; I was putting my hand in every other top hat I could find hoping to pull out a rabbit.

Facts: No new tumors, all the tumors were in the same place, they kept growing. Question: Could we do something localized? I remember my male friends with prostate cancer having radiation seeds implanted and I was wondering if we could do something like that. After a number of conversations with my medical oncologist, she agreed to refer me to a surgical oncologist to evaluate whether or not any of these more localized approaches might be possible.

It was quite a journey. Before we met, the surgical oncologist had looked at my file and become familiar with the particularities of my case and had let me know that they thought they would be able to help. My first face to face meeting was quite extraordinary. I have never had a physician discuss philosophies of treatment and my particular goals before. It seemed to me that it was crucial to this surgeon that I was aware and accepted that any surgical intervention would not be a cure, that I knew this disease was incurable. I appreciated our conversation immensely; I have never approached anything without being clear from a philosophical standpoint on the reasoning.

So, in addition to his multiple degrees and surgical oncology fellowship training and all of the rest of the paper trail that seems to indicate a skilled physician, the surgeon and I thought in holistic terms and were on the same wavelength. That was more important than I can convey, especially as I was trusting this man to cut out 35% of my lung tissue in an effort to improve the quality, and possibly the length of my life.

In May they operated on the least compromised lung. It was a minimally invasive surgery and I rebounded quickly. This, I thought, was going to be a snap and I felt guilty when I thought of my metavivor sisters (others with Stage 4 breast cancer) for whom this opportunity did not exist and who were wedded to traditional toxic chemo.

In June they operated on the more compromised lung. It was a full-blown thoracotomy where they cut off one entire lobe as well as a section of the remaining lobe. My ribs were fractured from having been spread, and while my skin was numb over a large portion of my chest, I had phenomenal nerve pain. Muscles were cut through and no longer functioned, not to mention that I felt like I was smothering. It was frightening, painful, and debilitating. I no longer felt guilty about having chosen an easier road than my metavivor sisters; I was paying the full load of suffering.

After five weeks it started to get better and I felt that I might actually be able to get past the pain. It has now been four months and I only have patches of numbness now, my muscles are starting to be useful once again, and I no longer gasp for air. I have gotten used to the feeling of not being able to breathe as deeply but I do get enough oxygen in every breath.

Three months after the surgery I went in for another scan to establish my new post-surgery baseline. I was expecting to have the scan look all shiny and new without the distinctive crab-like form of my former tumors. But, as with everything in cancer-land, a new suspicious lesion is now visible near where one of the tumors used to be. We won't know whether it is cancer or not, but I suspect that it is. The tumor site that it is near is the one tumor that never behaved no matter what we threw at it, the one that grew when all the others were shrinking.

Even if this new site is cancer, I have been able to reset the cancer clock. I hope that I have regained the 3 years that it took for the original metastases to grow to the size where they imperiled my life. I may have less time than that before I am back in the same situation as before, or I may have more time. With this disease you eventually learn not to hope and not to expect, just to take it as it comes.

But for now I have gained 10 pounds and have plump rosy

cheeks. When I look in the mirror I no longer see someone who is dying. I am living and loving. Life is full of surprises and adventures and is very, very good!

Healing vs. Cure

I am struggling with the meaning of healing. I am an introvert and never has this been more plain than the past few months. When I am stressed I withdraw and ponder and try to make meaning out of my situation. That is what we do as humans, make meaning, but extroverts make meaning out loud, with others. I just rabbit away until I can face the world again. I haven't been communicating with friends because I haven't known what to say. I was lost in this deep interior world trying to make meaning.

A few months ago I began to have difficulties associated with childhood polio. I would have days when I would not be able to walk, or days devoid of energy. For someone previously very active and in good physical condition, except for the cancer, this was difficult to accept. I had no control over my body and no sense of when my body would give up on me.

Shortly after I began to work with a physical therapist on this problem, I was told by my oncologist that my cancer tumors had started to grow again, that my treatment failed, and that we might have to consider another measure. I truly felt besieged. Maybe I could deal with one of these, but both at the same time? I wasn't so sure.

The physical therapist told me that I would not be able to ski this year. Skiing is my passion, it is what makes a winter in Montana worthwhile. It is liberating, but even more I sense God's presence in the silence of the snow and the power of the mountains. How can I survive winter without skiing?

When I was told that the cancer was growing again, I felt so foolish. I had just allowed my emotional defenses to relax, just allowed myself to begin to hope again after four months of my oncologist telling me and my husband that I was well. As soon as I was emotionally vulnerable again, the cancer reappeared. It is a very mean-spirited disease.

How does one find healing when there is no cure? As a health practitioner, I have often talked with my patients about healing and the difference between healing and cure, but I suppose it has been more of an abstraction for me until now. Neither of my conditions is curable so where is the healing for me? Healing is more than a positive mental attitude. I think that the process of healing involves going down into the muck of the illness in all its incarnations. It involves experiencing all of the ugliness, horror, and fear. But, after that, it also involves looking at it and saying, "That's OK. It is what it is, no more and no less."

For me it isn't about hope; what do I hope for? To be rid of these conditions? That's not going to happen. To have a good day? Some will be good and some not. It's about living in the moment, fully, with the negative and the positive and allowing each its rightful measure. Perhaps healing is acceptance in some way, not acceptance as in caving in to doom, but acceptance as in here you are and you are what you are, not more and not less.

My psychology professor had a wonderful way of expressing this. She told me to greet each thing that overwhelmed me by saying: "There you are. Please come in and let's have tea." Or another expression: "There you are. Have a seat on the bus. You can journey with me but you're not driving!"

So just maybe I have experienced healing. Maybe it means that to be healed doesn't mean being cheerful all of the time, or always thinking positively. Perhaps, it is as simple as facing disease and fear as they are but not more. I am not my diseases. I am.

I Can't Feel Good: I'll Disappoint My Friends!

One of the oddities of living with metastatic cancer is the investment that other people have in your illness. It is very strange. There is a woman I know who, when she sees me, will ask how I am. If I say I am fine, she will peer at me closely and probe further. If I continue to maintain that I feel fine, she will radiate disappointment. But, if I say that I am having a bad day she will beam with concern and well wishes and walk away seeming satisfied.

When I was first diagnosed with breast cancer, I reached out to my friends and they were marvelous. They responded with offers of transportation, food, watering my plants, and walking my dog and they kept offering for the year I was in treatment. When I was diagnosed with metastases to the lungs, I again reached out to my friends. They shared my grief and fear over the future. But then look what happened! The drama is gone and my cancer and I are just hanging out together like an old married couple. Where does that leave my friends?

For sure, when the tumors start to get rambunctious again, the drama will return but what do we do in the meantime? My friends have invested so much in supporting me. Where is the payoff for them in befriending a boring cancer patient? If I feel good, am I upsetting their expectations? What to do?

Living with this disease means long stretches of boredom punctuated by highlights of pure terror. It's hard on my friends to stay with me on this roller coaster. Is today a day when I feel like a well person or a sick person? It is the special friend who can take you as you are, support you when you need it, and treat you like a whole person regardless of where the roller coaster is at any given moment.

I am still someone living with Stage 4 breast cancer. (I don't feel I can call myself a survivor. Isn't that term for someone who has beaten the disease? I think that's one of those pink ribbon words.) Those of us in this situation are initiates into a dreadful secret society. And, while I have a tendency to freely share information, perhaps only other initiates should share in the intimate details of the Stage 4 experience, because only they truly grasp its long-term nature and gnarly twists and turns.

Perhaps it is enough that my friends know I have this terrible disease. More than that, perhaps it is enough that they know that I love them just as I know down into my bone marrow that they love me. Isn't that all that really matters?

Making a Decision But Fearing Its Consequences

A few months ago, after going back on chemo, I decided that I would not do any more chemo until the new stealth drugs are on the market. You see I am one of those pesky outliers, the ones that don't fit the statistical profiles and probabilities. After being on the threshold of death due to cancer treatment on more than one occasion, I decided that I would rather feel good on no treatment than feel bad and possibly die sooner because I was having cancer treatment, if that makes sense.

I am still convinced that my decision is the right one for me. I have been taking Herceptin alone since I discontinued the Xeloda two months ago. Statistically Herceptin is only 20% effective if it is not taken with a cytotoxic, but I am betting my life that it is the best course for me.

That being said, on Monday I will go into the CT scanner and learn what has been going on since I made this momentous decision. My tumor markers have never indicated that I have cancer, so the only way we know what is going on is through periodic scans. (I probably have enough radiation in me that if I don't die of this breast cancer I might from some later radiation induced one. It is such a paradox, this disease/treatment.) I am scared. I am scared that we might find the tumors have grown and that my life expectancy is dramatically reduced. I am scared because I have run out of options.

It is one thing to look death in the face when you have a treatment buffer between the two of you. I am afraid of what it is going to be to look death in the face when it is just the two of us. I am trying to tell myself that in reality nothing will have changed; I am still me, my life is still my life, my friends are still my friends. Yet, we will be totally changed in ways I can't and don't want to process yet.

As a behavioral scientist who has worked with cancer patients for many years I know what I have to do, I know what the tasks are before me. I have completed my life review. I am content that I am loved, that my life has had meaning, and that I have done work that has benefited the greater society. I have no regrets and nothing left undone. My "bucket" list is practically nonexistent. I have friends who have been touched by this disease before when loved ones have died; they know what lies ahead and they have promised that I won't be alone when the time comes. I am overwhelmingly blessed.

I also am overwhelmingly greedy! I love my life and I want more of it. I want to float down the river and catch a beautiful little cutthroat trout. I want to watch a Dutch oven turn over and spew its contents all over my driveway as my friends laugh. I want to explore the mountains more and communicate with the wild animals. I want to spare my friends the pain that will eventually come.

I'm not afraid of death. I am not so sanguine about dying of this horrible disease. But mostly I am afraid of having this amazing life that I worked hard all of my life to develop taken away, of not being able to share the wisdom that was so costly to acquire, of not being able to help heal others. As one patient said to me, I will miss being able to smell and touch and see and hear all the things this body makes possible.

I am confident in the decision that I made, but that does not mean that I get a free pass on the emotions that will result from its consequences.

Surviving and Catching Up

Time has flown by and I have been overwhelmed and very busy surviving. Those who do not think that surviving takes effort, focus, and determination, have never had cancer. I am amazed at how much energy it takes to just get through a day, and if that day has any kind of emotional upset you can almost just write off the next two or three.

A while ago I became convinced that I was going to die. I spent the next few months getting my head around that idea and becoming OK with the prospect. I continued with treatment but we were not expecting much in return and I turned my mind to accomplishing all of the things that I would need to do before my death.

My goddaughter, whom I love very much but see seldom, lives in Scotland. Other than my husband, she is my primary heir and it was important to me to see her one last time. So, I planned a wonderful trip to Scotland and a friend decided to join me. We went by ourselves, stayed in hostels, traveled on public transportation and used all of the money we saved to eat outrageously good meals.

About halfway through the trip I started feeling better. "Hmmm," I said to myself, "am I actually feeling better or is it because I am having such a good time?" When I got home I had some scans that found that most of my tumors had actually shrunk (except one delinquent that isn't minding anything we do to it). This was something I wasn't expecting and was totally unprepared for. So, the next few weeks were spent in trying to adjust to the idea of living. To adjust to the idea that there was, indeed, a faint possibility that I might actually outlive my husband. Things that I had been able to take in stride suddenly became annoying. My life seemed too small, I didn't seem to be doing all that I was capable of doing, perhaps I had made wrong choices recently that needed to be rethought.

All in all it was a very tumultuous time. As soon as I came to a place of relative tranquility I had my next scans. Well, whiplash isn't just an effect of car wrecks! The results were not good, nothing shrank, some things grew. Gone are the ideas of outliving my husband, replaced by the thought that I might really die within the next year or so.

In talking with my oncologist the only possibility for me now is to try another chemo agent. I swore that I would not do this, but now that the reality has come I am having to at least consider it again. I am truly in the odd place of, as one person said, fearing my treatment more than my disease. I think this is something unique to the cancer experience. I do fear it.

Every time I have been on chemo I have been a whisker from death. Even though this possible new agent is supposed to not affect most people, there is a distinctly high possibility that it will affect me, and the side effects include kidney failure and a remaining life on dialysis. Other treatments are awaiting that we have not considered because they damage the nerves and I already have damaged nerves from polio. Perhaps I could take them, but then I would spend the rest of my life in a wheelchair, unable to do most things that I love. [Postscript: I do have to add that since this was written I have had to revisit this again and again. Some things I said I would never accept I have come to placidly agree to in a trade off with death.]

I don't know what I will choose. I am taking time to make the decision and taking into consideration not only how much longer I might live with or without the drug but also the quality of my relationships and what I really want out of what is left of my life. I wish it wasn't all so confusing and tiring, but it is. There is no clear-cut path, no guaranteed route to success. There is only dogged perseverance, hope, and the self struggling to hold onto its dignity.

To Treat or Not to Treat: Questioning Life with Cancer

The last time I wrote I had just gotten the news that my cancer was growing again. The previous "soft" hormonal treatments were no longer working; it was time to bring out the big guns. My doctor and I went over all of the options and picked the chemotherapy agent that we thought would do the job with the least side effects. I was prepared to give it the old college try, even though I had once said that I would never go through chemo again, because I do want to live. I love my life and would like to keep it a bit longer. However, this new treatment had its own surprises and once again I have had to make decisions and go my own way.

I seem to be an outlier: every cytotoxin I have ever been on has tried to kill me. This time it was the Xeloda. After ten days of being on treatment I ended up in the hospital with every single side effect listed and then some. My GI tract was burned and blistered from mouth to bottom. I had hand/foot syndrome, massive explosive diarrhea and subsequent dehydration, phenomenal gut pain, an infection they could never identify but that Cipro knocked out, and a fungal infection on my skin. I was also anemic and my ketones and liver function tests were off the charts.

I was in the hospital for seven days before they would trust me to come home. Eating was a torture but I worked my way up from fats and meats to whole grain. Once I mastered them I got to move on to cooked veggies. Yahoo!

The upshot of all of this is that I felt that I needed to review the options available to me. I decided that I will not do traditional chemo anymore. I will continue on with Herceptin, but I will steer clear of the traditional cytotoxins.

This has been a decision that has been hard on my friends and family. We are so bought into the scientific studies of treatment outcomes that we forget that the science really only works on a bell curve. If you have someone like me who does not fit within the bell, you really don't know what treatment is going to do.

I am convinced now that if I do traditional treatment, it will not just make me miserable, it will kill me. So I have decided to take my chances on feeling better for whatever time I have left. It may be short or long, but at least I won't be in the hospital wishing I was dead already. My husband supports me in this although it has raised a lot of emotions for him that I think he would prefer not to deal with.

We won't know what this decision means in terms of my longevity until I have my next scans so we are living in limbo to some extent, but we are intentionally living each moment and that is the point.

Journal Entries: Daily Life with Metastatic Disease

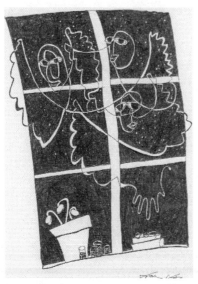

Daily life with metastatic cancer feels like stretches of extreme boredom interspersed with moments of chilling fear. The types of boredom are usually the same, the merry-go-round of doctors' appointments, scans, labwork, and procedures. If I didn't have cancer I wouldn't have a social life; all of my interpersonal conversations take place in the doctor's office, and I consider the doctors and nurses as friends! Some weeks I have three different appointments and two different sets of scans. Cancer has become my profession, as much as I did not want it to. But the fear is different each time. When you are first diagnosed the fear is related to having scans and getting the results. You are so afraid that the news is going to be bad news because you just know you are going to die at any minute. After you have lived with the disease for a few years, the fear lessens. You know you are most likely not going to die tomorrow, and so you are a bit more chill. That lasts until the results that you receive are not good ones. In the face of worsening disease the icy fingers of fear grab you around the throat; you try to relax but you really don't want to die.

It seems like cancer laughs at you. As soon as I would finally be able to release the fear, and trust that the tests were right and things were getting better, that is when things inevitably got worse. This happens so often that eventually you come to terms with it somehow: it may get better, it may get worse, ho hum, today's a nice day. When you get to the stage where I am now, you know it isn't getting any better and that you have run out of options. I find that now I am trying to live in the face of death while holding this knowledge lightly. It is a little bit like having come full circle but having lost the reactive bits.

So, what follows are excerpts from my journal. I have included them to take you with me on this roller-coaster ride. They are not dated, as the dates are meaningless, but they are offered in chronological order over the seven or so years from the point that the first metastatic tumor was found in my lung until the last excerpt which was written a few weeks ago. You will notice that my attitude changes and that my coping skills change; sometimes I seem fine with everything and sometimes I am overwhelmed. Sometimes it seems that emotionally and spiritually I am spinning in circles. That chaos is life with cancer, it just is. No one ever masters it, we all just do the best we can.

* * * *

So here's the deal. After almost five years of thinking I was cancer free, I recently found that my breast cancer actually spread and I now have Stage 4 breast cancer with metastases to the lung and possibly the bone. At times I am overwhelmed with the news but mostly I am so happy that it was found early, and quite by accident. If it had not been for my very bad dog running after some wildlife while we were hiking, I would not have fallen and not had an x-ray to see if I had broken a rib. That is when the tumor was spotted.

The metastases have been there since my original diagnosis, and were clearly only marginally affected by my original chemo and ongoing hormone therapy. That's kind of creepy. But they have been held back so that they are only now becoming large enough to see in the scans.

This is going to be a very different experience because I will be fighting this battle for the rest of my life. Hence, it is not going to be a few months of acute anguish and then we are done. It is going to be a slow and ultimately boring process. So please be patient with me. There will be times when nothing is going on (which is a very good thing) and there will be times when we find that a treatment is no longer working which will result in intense reflections.

I do not know how this is going to play out, but I do believe in the power of prayer and in the Holy Spirit. My life is in God's hands.

* * * *

The path lab is going to be running another panel on the tumor material they retrieved during the biopsy to try and get an exact profile of the tumor so we can tailor treatment accordingly. The oncologist believes that we can treat this with hormone therapy and save chemo for down the road when we may need it. This is fine for me as I will be able to continue my normal activities and be able to ski and ride horses through the winter months. In the interim, she has taken me off of Arimidex, which I have taken for the past 4 years, and put me on tamoxifen. While Arimidex is the state of the art anti-estrogen drug, it hasn't completely been successful so we will try others to see if they work better for me. My original tumor was HER2 receptor positive. We are hoping that this material is as well (the doc says that the tumor profile can change over time). If it is, then we have a powerful weapon in Herceptin.

So, I am going to enjoy this absolutely gorgeous Montana fall day, and thank God for the privilege of being here. Later we are going to go for a short hike, but without the dog!

I am overwhelmed by the love that has poured out to me since this diagnosis. What an amazing group of friends I have. Many of the kind words shared with me have given me the assurance that my life has not been in vain and that if it ends shortly I will leave this earth having touched the lives of others in a positive way and having served God as well as I have been able.

* * * *

I have been thinking the past few days about this cancer and how I should respond to it. When I was first diagnosed with cancer I took this very accepting "cancer as friend" approach. And, while the cancer certainly taught me many important lessons and changed my life for the better, my approach clearly did nothing in terms of getting rid of it for good. So, I now think that perhaps looking at it as a foreign pest might be more efficacious. For a while I started calling the tumors "Hannigan" after Miss Hannigan in Annie, because she was a bully and a coward who beat up on little orphans. But it didn't seem an easy fit.

The image that has come to mind and lodged there is that the tumors are cockroaches. You know the saying that cockroaches are probably going to be the only thing that survives a nuclear holocaust? Well, these suckers survived a chemo that came within an eyelash of killing me. They are little things that have skittered everywhere in my lungs; I think it is an apt analogy to having lived in an apartment house that had a terrible cockroach problem. You fight them, they skitter away. Later they skitter on back and you fight them again. Sort of like this stage of cancer. Well, that is my wisdom for today. My doctor just called and my bloodwork was normal, no elevation in tumor markers (what a crafty disease)! And, as I am reclaiming my life from this disease I am off to the health club to work out. It feels great to be able to work my body in spite of the roaches.

* * * *

I just returned from my bone scan. I checked online to see what normal looks like so I would know a bit more about what I saw. These results are merely what I saw on the screen as I lay in the scanner. It appears that I may have some involvement in my ribs, unless it was picking up the costochondritis that is there. I also lit up in my shins and in my feet, particularly one foot, although that could be arthritis and an old injury. I have no idea about my head and neck since I was inside the scanner and could not see the monitor. So I have to wait for the results on Tuesday, and pray for the best. They shouldn't let patients see the monitor, it just scares us. It looks like something and could easily be nothing. So I am trying to settle myself after thinking that things might be a lot worse. Now that I have thought it through, I don't think it is as bad as all that, so I now have to work off the adrenaline and recapture my balance.

* * * *

Well, finally I have good news to share. All of my angst over the bone scan turned out to be about nothing, just as I surmised after I had calmed down enough to be able to actually think. All of the places that lit up on the bone scan were due to arthritis and other causes. I have no bone mets. Yea! The tumor panel showed that the cancer is still HER2 positive which means that we will be able to use Herceptin when the time comes. However, the oncologist does not think that time is now. She is waiting to see what the tamoxifen does. If it works then that is all I will need to do for the time being. If it doesn't work then we will try something else. It will take the tamoxifen a month to get up to full strength in my system, so I am to see her in a month. If my symptoms worsen in the meantime I am to go in to be checked right away. Thanks for the prayers! They are making a difference. My job for now is to learn how to live with the cockroaches and not freak out. Blessings to all.

* * * *

Well, as I said before, no news is good news. I haven't written because there really isn't anything new to tell. I see the oncologist on December 3. I suspect that I won't have scans until sometime in January. I feel fantastic. I have been going to the gym religiously every day and working out for 90 minutes. The research on the beneficial aspects of exercise on breast cancer is really compelling. While I didn't heed it in the past, it has become the way I can try and fight these roaches now, and I am quite diligent. It is so odd having this lethal disease and yet feeling wonderful. It is like consciously living and dying simultaneously.

One thing that I have found is that there are not many resources for women with metastatic disease. The vast majority of information and resources are aimed at the newly diagnosed, or people going through adjuvant therapy. I have not been able to find any resources, with the exception of the Metastatic Breast Cancer Network, that help me cope with living in this strange space.

Apparently other women in my position are finding the same thing and there is the beginning of a movement to get cancer publications and conferences to include information specifically for those of us who belie the happy "Rah, Rah, Beat Cancer" tone of so much of what is out there. We will never beat cancer; we can only hope to keep it at bay long enough to die of something else. It may be that the general population doesn't want to know that we exist because it heightens fears about treatment not working. But I believe that it is important, not only for us to have a presence, but for others to know that it is possible to live with this disease for many, many years. If I didn't have a couple of friends here who have been living with metastatic disease for a number of years, and whose wisdom makes it possible for me to have hope and to live my life, I don't know how I might be reacting to this.

The Metastatic Network site has a statistic that says that 25% of breast cancer patients have these cancer "seeds" (what I am calling my roaches). These are cells that have migrated from the original tumor and seeded someplace else and withstood the original treatment only to pop up later. Who knew? So the watchword for now is to really live! Blessings to all!

* * * *

I hope that all of you had a happy Thanksgiving. Bill and I had our Thanksgiving dinner at a local resort sitting by a lake with a beautiful sunset and a crackling fire in the fireplace. We reflected on and off through the meal about all that we have to be thankful for. Truly we are very blessed.

While I am very aware of my blessings, the emotional part of this situation beat down on me last weekend as I had a couple of teary days and one small panic attack recalling the mind-numbing fear I felt on the day I had my bone scan. While I am prepared for death, I don't want to die. I had lunch with our wonderful priest on Monday and she helped get me back in balance again. Her personal take on it is that God has called me to Montana, specifically for a ministry at St. Pat's and she sees me being there for a long time. In line with that, we are starting a healing ministry tomorrow at the church. That was one of my primary ministries before we moved and so I am delighted to be able to start something up here. We shall see how it goes and, if there is enough interest, we may continue a mid-week healing service after Christmas.

Meanwhile, I need to rev up the old spiritual discipline. Funny how you know things but conveniently forget them from time to time. When I met with our priest I was reminded of a visit to my spiritual director once when she asked me quite bluntly, "Why, are you here? You know what you need to do, so go do it." Nothing like being a caregiver and completely ignoring the advice you give to everyone else! I will write again after I see my oncologist later next week. May you have a peace-filled and joyful holiday season surrounded by friends and loved ones.

* * * *

The meeting with the oncologist went well. There is a possibility for a drug interaction between the tamoxifen and another medicine that I am taking, so she ordered some blood tests to see how I metabolize the tam' as well as a standard panel. I have my next scan scheduled for Jan. 5 and my follow-up appointment with the oncologist on Jan. 7.

I am very eager for this because it will be the first time we will have any indication whether this treatment is effective or whether we will need to try something else. Fingers crossed! Meanwhile, I know the tam' is working because I have never had so many hot flashes in my life. It's like I am about to spontaneously combust at any moment. It's great to be in Montana because at least I can walk outside when it gets too bad. I guess it is a small price to pay if it works and I can keep skiing, etc. this winter but it certainly is a bother and uncomfortable.

So unless something comes up or I am the victim of some Deep Thought, I will write again next month when I have more news. Happy Holidays, Merry Christmas, many blessings!

* * * *

We have moved my scans up a couple of weeks and I will be having them this Friday afternoon. I will then see my oncologist a week from today, Tuesday. My doc has just returned from the breast cancer conference and looked over my labs. According to the lab report I should metabolize the tam' very well but we don't know what impact another medicine may be having on this (apparently it interferes with the process). So, she has moved the scans up so we can see how well it is working. Meanwhile, I have titrated myself off of the other medicine and hope that will help. While that medicine was once very important, I believe that our change in circumstances has had salient benefits and that this other particular medicine is not so critical now.

So, what we are hoping for is that things are stable. It may be a bit early to see much shrinkage in the tumors, but if the meds are not working we would definitely see growth. I will write next week after I have seen the doctor. What a lovely Christmas present it would be to have a good report. Of course, the initial diagnosis was my Christmas present five years ago. This is a time of wonder and mystery and seems appropriate. Blessings!

* * * *

I just returned from seeing my oncologist and getting the results of my scans. The disease is stable, meaning that none of the cockroaches has gotten any larger (although they are not any smaller either). This is apparently my new normal.

An interesting thing I learned today is that carcinomas have a shell around them and the cell can be dead but the shell will still show up on a scan until the body begins to absorb it, unlike some others where the cancer just melts away. We still have a problem with drug interactions and haven't figured out how to solve it but so far the treatment seems to be holding things stable regardless. So, we are going to continue with the treatment for now. My next scan will be the last week of February unless my symptoms worsen, in which case I see her immediately. I have been quite contemplative today. My surgery was exactly five years ago today. What an experience! Merry Christmas!

* * * *

Nothing momentous to add. I am feeling great. Had a little blip

where people were trying to be helpful and ended up trans-
ferring their own anxiety about breast cancer to me. But, if I hold
on to my own North Star, I am very peaceful about it all for now.

I have a great doc who is tailoring my treatment to the specific
needs of my body. She is not worried at this point, so I am taking
my cues from her. A friend of mine, who is a doc and an expert in
women's health, recently visited us here in Montana. She stressed
to me that it isn't the cells that are in one's body that should be a
source of concern, it is what one's body is doing with those cells.

So for now, the cockroaches are just hanging out, no biggie. I
have no symptoms and have been able to get out and ski. Yahoo!
I am still working out at the fitness center every day. I have even
started working on writing a new book. Yowza.

For Christmas a friend gave me a gift under the Cancer Vixen
label. I had not heard of this book, but when I looked it up I
thought it was fabulous. It is a graphic novel about a woman's
experience with breast cancer. The gist of it is how to kick
cancer's butt wearing four inch heels. I love it! In one acquain-
tance's terminology, it is definitely not kumbaya!

* * * *

There is this great song I want to share with everyone. It has
taken me a while to get the details down. For years I thought it
had been recorded by Calaveras, a group based in the San
Francisco Bay Area, but Greg Beattie, blessed band member and
lawyer extraordinaire, just informed me that it was actually
written by Elaine Dempsey (who has graciously given her
permission for me to reproduce the lyrics below) and recorded by
a group now known as Big Wide Grin (then known as Elaine,
Lambert, and Karl) and recorded on an album named *Live Simple,
Breathe Deep*.

After this I'm gonna see Jamaica

After this I'm gonna dance and carry on
After this I'm gonna care less often
After this I'll be with you where I belong

After this I'm gonna linger longer
After this I'm gonna kiss this job goodbye
After this I'm gonna journey farther
After this I'm gonna be there by your side

With time for words
with time to hear what's on your mind
with time to shoulder all your cares
with time to solve all of the problems of the world
in time you'll know I will be there

After this I'm gonna dine on lobster
After this I'm gonna drink the finest wine
After this I'm gonna splurge on nonsense
After this I'm gonna savor wasted time

After this I'm gonna lose my bearings
After this I will surrender to your charms
After this I'm gonna love you better
After this I'm gonna wake up in your arms.

With time for passion
with time for matters of the heart
with time to idle all the while
with time for whispers from the one I've come to love
in time we'll make a life worthwhile
After this... After this... After this... After this...

Life carries on, before you know it things have gone
another promise swiftly flies

age calls me quickly as the years roll on and on
and you're still here right here by my side
Well, after this (you know I'll get around to you, honey)
After this (just think Jamaica)
After this... After this...

* * * *

Friends have been e-mailing and expressing concern that I haven't written in awhile. Not to worry. No news is good news. My next scans are on Friday and I will write after I get the results. Meanwhile, I have had a really bad respiratory infection for the past three weeks. We went to Park City for a long awaited ski vacation with friends and, after a half day of skiing, I spent the entire time in bed coughing and sniffling. I finally went to the doctor today just as a precaution and she has put me on Z-Pak. She is not worried though and thinks that this should resolve in time. My concern is that I don't want to pay the $2,000 (or have my insurance company pay it) for the scan and find out the results are messed up because of this infection.

One thing of interest I did learn today is that having lung mets makes you more susceptible to bacterial lung infection. Good thing to know.

It is a gorgeous day. Bright sun and clear sky. They are holding a dog ski-joring race in West Glacier and if I can stand the cold dry air we are going to try and go for a little while. I'll let everyone know my scan results probably in ten days or so. Blessings!

* * * *

Just a quick note. I saw my oncologist today. The results of the scans were satisfactory but not great. The tumors are still there and haven't shrunk. On the other hand, they haven't grown either. My doctor said she would feel better if they had shrunk. However, she also said that with my aggressive cancer she believes that the medicine must be working or she feels the tumors would have grown. I am to see her again in six weeks and then we will decide where to go from here. I am pleased in general. I would have liked for the tumors to have shrunk as well but I'll take stable.

My quality of life is still very good. I went skiing today and had a wonderful time. That is the main thing for me right now. I read today that the average life expectancy for metastatic breast cancer is two years. I have been stable for four months now so I am hoping that I will beat that statistic!

* * * *

I have been trying to decide what to write about the last few weeks. You see, I am not this strong upbeat person all of the time and a couple of weeks ago I had an absolute tsunami of terror engulf me. I had allowed myself to get a little too stressed. There were some complications with my medicines as well. In the midst of this I allowed myself to read some statistics regarding the average life expectancy of someone in my situation and the average efficacy period for any drug used to treat the disease. Needless to say, the stats were shocking and threw me into a tailspin. If I hadn't been tired and stressed to begin with I might have been able to parse through the data with what I know to be my particular factors, but I wasn't, and I couldn't, so I didn't.

One fortunate thing to come out of all of this is that Bill and I are now really talking about what I want, what will happen to him if I die, etc. It has been a relief not to have to keep a brave face on in front of each other and to be able to be authentic about what lies ahead. I take comfort in the knowledge that these cancer seeds have been in my body for over six years. The fact that they are still tiny is a major victory given how aggressive my cancer is.

I have tremendous support from friends here in the valley as well as friends elsewhere. I have an excellent oncologist. I am learning how to take things as they come and not "borrow trouble" (as my grandmother used to say). But it is not an easy lesson and I keep having to have refresher courses! One thing I have discerned is that I am not afraid of death but I am afraid of the dying process, particularly with cancer. But when, and if, that comes it will be down the road. The sun is shining and I have my knitting to get back to! Blessings.

* * * *

Saw my oncologist today. Other than my reactive airways due to a long drawn out case of bronchitis earlier this year, and a new respiratory infection that is going around the valley, I seem to be doing well. She does not think that the cancer is doing anything other than hanging out. Especially since I am able to be so physically active. I am due to have another CT scan in early May and to see her again shortly afterwards. They also did bloodwork today, the first time in three months or so. So we shall see what's what at the next appointment.

My doc is amazed that the cancer isn't doing anything after all of this time. As aggressive as my cancer is, it is quite something that it is just hanging out. I attribute it to all of the prayers that are going up and have gone up for me and this situation. Thank God! Blessings to all of you dear friends who are on this journey with me by choice and in love. I'll write next month after I get my results back.

* * * *

Saw my oncologist today to get the results of the CT I had last week. The tumors are unchanged. The doc said that she would feel better if they would shrink but, given the fact that at one point they clearly were growing, the fact that they are unchanged and that my symptom load is light, she will take stable as a good thing. I think she has given up on the idea that we might ever get these things to go away so I need to get used to having them just hanging out. We are going to ride out this treatment course as long as we can, that is until the tumors start to grow again. When they start growing we will see what we do next.

There are lots of options available, some much less pleasant than others. The treatment course I am on now is the easiest and least compromising in terms of quality of life which is one reason we are staying with it. I also don't want to use up my options too quickly. So I see her again in six weeks.

Still trying to wrap my head around just who I am with this disease. Having it makes me hyper-vigilant which I hate. But if I don't pay attention to subtle signals this cancer will take me over before I know what hit me. Bill and I were talking a couple of days ago. He is confused and doesn't know whether to treat me like a sick person or a well person. I am confused because I don't know whether I consider myself a sick person or a well person. At times my self-concept changes multiple times a day. Not exactly easy to live with and very difficult to try and make plans because I may have to bail on them. Trying to get to a place of acceptance but not there yet. Hope Dame Julian was right when she said that all shall be well and all manner of thing shall be well. Right now just really bummed.

* * * *

A friend and fellow chaplain and I have been engaged in an e-mail dialog since I last wrote. It has helped clarify my thoughts and I wanted to share them with you now. Here is the dialog; the text in quotes is my friend's contribution.

"[We] were talking at lunch today about how we both were so

grateful to you for your sharing about your experiences and how what you were saying informed our own chaplaincy efforts. I do hope you know how very much we, and I'm sure many others, appreciate what you are telling us about what it's like from inside."

Thanks for the feedback. That is my intention, that by sharing I can help shed some light and bring about deeper understanding. Of course, as with any chronic disease, some of my friends just wish I would stop puling and get on with my life!

"We were wondering about how you feel about your cancer. That is, is the cancer that you tell us is in your body to stay 'me' the way, say, your little finger is, or is it 'not me'? The origin of this question is your comment about wondering how to think of yourself, as 'sick' or as 'well.' So are you the cancer, or is the cancer simply a part of you, or is the cancer something you reject even though you can't, really, or is there some entirely different formulation?"

I woke up this morning at 5:00am with this question ringing in my mind. Of course, as we know, the mere asking of a question changes the dynamics and may have therapeutic effect, so bless you both! I believe this question is the crux of the matter and I have been too close to see it. I have been viewing the cancer as Other, as "not me." When I went through treatment the first time, I saw it as Other but a benevolent Other, sort of like a medical angel that had been sent into my life to teach me some life lessons.

That is all very well and good when you have the expectation that treatment, however horrific, will be successful and once you have learned your lesson the little guys will go away and never visit again. Belleruth Naparstek, in her wonderful cancer visualization tapes, has a part where you thank your cancer and tell it that it can go now, that you understand what it was sent to tell you. So I was very intent, as you may remember, on learning my lesson and being grateful to my cancer.

This situation really challenges that approach. There is all sorts of room for self-recrimination: Was I not grateful enough? Did I not learn the lesson I was to learn? And on and on. It is made a little worse when I am told that the treatment that almost killed me did not, in fact, kill the cancer and that these buggers have been around in hiding all of that time.

What struck me during my sleep, and floated into consciousness upon waking, is that this dichotomy between other and self is in fact the source of my psychological and spiritual distress. If I turn it around and say that these cancer cells are part of Me (not "me" as there is a vast difference) then the tension dissolves. As a doctor friend of mine keeps reminding me, it is not the cells in my body but what my body does with the cells that should concern me. So I believe that a more helpful view is that these cancer cells are the physical equivalent to the psyche's Shadow.

Now taking that view opens up all sorts of new avenues for wholeness. As someone who is used to living in my head, the physical self has been the dumping ground for all of those things that I wanted to ignore or reject. My solid grounding in evangelical Protestant thought has set me up for the spirit:good::body:evil mindset, and even though I am an Anglican now with Druidic Celtic tones and mentally reject such nonsense, that upbringing is deep in my unconscious. I know from my work that the Shadow is a fertile ground for spiritual work and that when we are open to our Shadow-selves God speaks to us with great power.

"As you know from your spiritual and psychological work, the usual teaching is that if we deny our pain, or fear or wound-edness or whatever, we give it strength, while if we lean into it we metabolize it and are less caught up in it. But does this apply to a physical situation like yours?"

I have not been denying my woundedness (in fact some friends recently wrote and told me that I should be "divorcing" this cancer and quit focusing on it so much) but that appears to have given it more power. It is not the denial or acceptance, for either can be deadly. One can deny to one's peril as we know, but one can also accept it in a passive way that also insures dire consequences so I don't think that that formula is exactly applicable in this situation.

If I were to deny this cancer, while I am in the middle of an asthma attack that is a direct result of the tumors' presence, that is stupid and dangerous. Likewise, if I just say that that's the way it is, and don't pay attention, then that is also stupid and dangerous as my cancer is the most aggressive form (next to inflammatory) of breast cancer. I don't think metabolizing is the right verb either. I think that approaching this as one does one's Shadow, seeing what is there, what is fearful, etc. but accepting that this too is part of who one is, and then striving to learn from its wisdom. The fear is real, the physical discomfort is real, the danger is real but... I must learn to love all of my cells.

For years, as the physical shadow, my body was a source of disappointment and a reminder of trauma and shame. I have only recently been able to look at my body and all that it has been through and realize what a wonderful body it is and how it has fought so valiantly for my well-being in spite of disrespect and disregard. Even when the cancer was discovered, I was struck by how my body had been able to not let the disease completely overrun me and, while I got a big honking tumor that scared the bejeesus out of the doctors in under 6 months' time, there was no evidence of it in my lymph nodes and only the one discernable tumor.

So I am coming to a place where I believe I will be able to trust my body with these tumors as well. As with our psyches, the Shadow in my body presents things to me that I must pay attention to but have succeeded in banishing from my consciousness: when to get enough rest, when to get out of situations because they are too stressful, etc. So intentional engagement with it can be a powerful source of healing (though not necessarily cure). I cannot thank you enough for being willing to enter into dialogue with me and to help me process this.

* * * *

I can't believe that today marks our one year anniversary in the valley! The year, though not exactly what we had envisioned, has born testament to the rightness of my desire to be here. In spite of the new(ish now) diagnosis of Stage 4 and attendant pulmonary infections and the fact that I am now typing this one handed as the other hand (broken while on the trail) lies around basking in the novelty of its new, very hi-tech, titanium plate and screws hiding beneath a quite stylish soft cast, my quality of life is very, very good indeed. I am where I want to be and able to be quite comfortable in my own skin at long last.

Another friend, from the Washington on the western coast, has also entered into this dialogue which has gone on between me and my East Coast chaplain friends. Julie's insights have helped to deepen my self-awareness. Her understanding is that cancer cells are mostly normal cells that have no limit to growth and so run amok in our bodies commandeering nutrients and confounding our immune responses. She wonders if another way to look at this is as cells that developed in response to some unknown assaults but that have stayed on past their usefulness. She likens this to 12-step programs that refer to childhood coping mechanisms that are no longer adaptive when we are adults. This struck me as being an interesting level of inquiry.

I believe that it is possible that these cells grew in the presence of threats to my essential self, not to my physical body self but to the core of who I truly am; the exact same type of psychological and spiritual threats were battering me prior to both the original diagnosis and the subsequent discovery of the mets. These forces shared a common denominator: that my duty, and what I thought was my security, could only be achieved by obliterating my individual self in the service of others whom I had sworn before God and the company of saints to love. (Love here being an active verb not a romantic feeling.)

Perhaps these tumors were a metaphorical "not so fast!" Perhaps they were trying to insure that "I" lived on. They certainly gave me permission in society's eyes to focus on myself and what I wanted or needed. It also fits one of my long-held beliefs in the metaphorical power of illness. People react uncomfortably when they hear me say that I am not surprised that my cancer is breast cancer because I had so many people hanging onto my tits my whole life. (Ooh, she said "tits"! or "Well isn't that why women have them? They're supposed to be nurturers, for God's sake!") But that is my bodily understanding.

An aside here: how impoverishing is a world view that identifies our worth and meaning based upon whether we have wombs or penises, or whether our role is to nurture or to screw people. In such a world the screwers can't relent and the nurturers just get screwed. From a metaphorical point of view, I don't find it all that strange that men are seeing similar rises in prostate cancer. It may be that men aren't all that comfortable with the role of first and foremost having to screw things whether in business negotiations, sports, or relationships. But that's a subject for another day!

It could be that these cells were growing so rapidly in the face of soul sucking forces to keep me balanced in some weird metaphysical way. I, and my component parts, were doing the best we could with the information and experience at hand in the midst of unimaginable stress, and I am someone who grew up with stress as thick in the atmosphere as oxygen, so this was pretty bad. I wasn't able to understand at those times that the information and experience upon which I was relying was maladaptive. So from a deep shadowy place, it may be that this primitive knowledge about the nature of life and death inserted itself and these defiant cells responded to the threat. Weird, maybe, but worth thinking about a bit more. Blessings! Life is good!

* * * *

Saw my oncologist today. We addressed the problem of the drug interactions and, after discussing it with all of the doctors involved, we have decided that I will change off the antide pressant that reduces the tamoxifen's effectiveness. We thought we had it solved before by titrating off one of the medications but then a new study came out that implicated the one I remained on. So, here's hoping the antidepressants that are available to me are effective. If not then I will go back on the existing treatment and the cancer treatment will have to change.

My oncologist reminded me that we are going to have to change off the tamoxifen at some point because my cancer will adjust to it. We just don't know when that will be – in a year or five years or… I don't like thinking about it because this is so easy and I can fool myself into thinking that my disease is not so serious. We have scheduled my next CT scan for the end of July. We shall see what the roaches have been up to then.

* * * *

Well, friends, no news yet. I had my scans last Monday as planned but immediately was felled by a virus with high fever and horrific aches. I had to reschedule my oncology appointment until August 9 in order to get the results. I am taking it that nothing significant has changed or the doctor would have wanted to at least talk with me by telephone. So I will write again after August 9. Hope you are all having a happy summer. We have had lovely weather and the blessing of many friends visiting; it doesn't get much better than that!

* * * *

It just may be that a miracle has occurred. I saw my oncologist this morning and she told me that my scans are unchanged, but all my vitals are good as is my bloodwork. She is of the opinion that the tumors are dead. Carcinomas, as I have mentioned before, have a shell or carapace around them. The cancer can die as a result of treatment but the carapace will continue to be evident in scans until the body has had a chance to break it down and absorb it. Since my condition has been unchanged for ten months, she feels free to venture this informed opinion. It is so much more than I had hoped for. She is still going to monitor me for the next few months just to make sure but overall she told Bill that I was well! I feel like fizzy bubbles are shooting all throughout my body. So, I have another reprieve. Who knows how long it will last but I will take it.

I am also convinced that being in a healing place, having fun, and amazing prayer support have all had a part to play in this. The key now is to keep doing what I have been doing and to make sure that I get enough rest every day and continue to live life fully and intentionally. I will probably not write again until I have seen my oncologist in two months. That is, of course, unless I have Deep Thoughts to share (remember the *Saturday Night Live* sketches? I always thought they were a hoot, especially as I am given to having deep thoughts).

Yesterday, God gave me a great birthday present. (My birthday was last week but this got started on my birthday.) I went fly-fishing on a float trip with some new friends. We had the absolutely perfect day: good weather, lots of fish, lots of laughter, great company and ending with warm huckleberry cobbler à la mode. Life is good!

* * * *

Well, friends, here is another wrinkle. It just seems that God does not want to cut me a break on this physical stuff. After that good news about the cancer, I now am having problems that may be related to the polio I had as a kid. An interesting aside, in 1955 the Salk vaccine was approved for general use after clinical tests. Unfortunately, approximately 260 children contracted polio from the vaccine and 10 of those died. (They also had a scary thing happen when in Denver 1,000 children were found to have become carriers of the polio virus and members of their families were becoming infected.) I was one of the lucky 250 kids who didn't die but did come down with the disease from the vaccine.

It has been a puzzling summer as I have had all sorts of things going on that might have been attributable to the cancer but now clearly are not. I have been having problems with fatigue but more than that my gait is affected, as is my balance, and I have been falling in certain situations. Some days I have had to walk with a cane and some days I haven't been able to walk at all as my legs would not carry my weight. In consulting the post-polio society Web site I learned that Post-polio Syndrome can come on after trauma, surgery, or periods of inactivity. Well, I had a traumatic fall earlier in the summer where I tore my hand an inch off my wrist (slipped to one side), which was followed by surgery and a period of inactivity. So... I have seen my primary care doctor and she has referred me to a neurologist, just to rule out anything else that might be causing this. The neurologist has a long waiting list so it will be about six weeks before I can get in to see him. I will write back here as soon as I have seen him and know anything else of interest.

On the positive side, I have found a warm water exercise class that doesn't stress my legs but gives me a good conditioning workout. Yea! And, our fishing has now transitioned from float trips on rivers, where I have had to stand up to fish for the most part, to lake fishing where I am in my own little pontoon boat or a belly boat and so can fish while sitting down. So I hope the class will add to my endurance and ability to stay out longer. Don't even want to think about what this may mean for ski season, especially as I have my new season pass in hand burning a hole in my pocket! So prayers for patience and prayers for hope are greatly needed. Thanks! Blessings too!

* * * *

Saw the neurologist today. Liked him very much. He ruled out all of the really bad things that could be going on. Yahoo! So for now he has me seeing a physical therapist. I start with her next Tuesday afternoon and we shall see whether this has any impact. I am hoping that it will. Meanwhile, I continue to moderate my activity and the rest is doing me worlds of good. It could be that I just plum overdid (who, me?) this past year and it caught up with me. I don't like the fact that my recent brush with metastatic cancer has turned me into Chicken Little. Guess that's what happens when you really want to live and are so afraid of life being snatched away. Thanks for the prayers, they have really helped.

* * * *

I had a good meeting with the Physical Therapist yesterday. Lots of tests and more to come. They are still trying to figure out what is going on with me. At this point in time, she says that post-polio is high on her list of suspects but that she is continuing to check for other potential factors. More tests to come on Thursday. She wants me to have my oncologist order a scan of my thoracic region just to rule out a bone met around T7. I feel good about this though; I think she is really going to be able to help nail down what is happening and what my limitations are. She seems to know a lot about polio and how it works and how it presents itself. Haven't had anyone take a look at this since I was 7 so it feels liberating to be able to talk about it and learn more about my particular situation. I have forgotten so much. Learned yesterday that one leg is shorter than the other as well as one leg being weaker than the other. Hmmm, do I see orthotics in my future? Updates to come.

* * * *

Saw my oncologist today to get results of my recent scans and MRI. The MRI of my spine was clear, which we expected, but the CT scans indicated that the tumors might be growing again. However, they were not definitive so I have to have another CT in six weeks to confirm these results. For the time being we are not changing medications until we know for sure that the tamoxifen is no longer effective. Too much going on physically. I am overwhelmed right now. I will write again in January. Meanwhile, have a wonderful holiday season.

* * * *

It seems my mets are growing again. We will try Faslodex to see if we can stay on endocrine treatments a little bit longer. If it does not work, I will have to go back on chemo again. I am angrier about this cancer than I have ever been! This outbreak has caused me to have to cancel a three-week trip to see very good friends that mean the world to me. Instead I have to stay here and get injections and have tests and jump through hoops and tag bases. Next stop is making sure the insurance company will pay for the drug and then scans to see if it has spread to other organs. I will write more when there is news.

* * * *

Saw my oncologist today. I had a chance to talk about all of the things that I have been pondering over the past months. The Faslodex takes a long time to work so the symptoms that I have been feeling are normal. The fact that they are easing somewhat now is a good sign. I will have my first scans since changing medications in early April. By then the drug should have had a long enough time to show us whether it will work or not. After Faslodex we are not going to try the taxanes, due to my post-polio neurological deficits. But I have been assured that there are plenty of other treatments out there to choose from, including two new ones that should be approved by the FDA at end of the month. My doctor said that the treatment I already had initially, AC, was as bad as it gets in terms of side effects and that she doesn't anticipate that any treatment I receive going forward will be as debilitating. That takes some of the sting out of all of this and I have renewed confidence that I will be able to manage.

I do tend to think I know definitively what is going on in my body, and sometimes I do but sometimes I really don't. I just had a humorous reminder of that, just in time. I broke my ankle a week ago. I spent three days telling everyone it was just a sprain. Finally, with my foot every color of the rainbow, but mostly jungle camo with accents of burgundy here and there, I went to the ortho who told me it was broken. So now I'm getting so much trash talk about being Dr. Vance (and not in the PhD sense)! It's been a good lesson that I can guess what is going on with this cancer, but I won't ever really know, and oftentimes I am wrong about what it is or how serious it may be. I'll fill you in in April after I get my scans back. But for now, the sun is out; spring is headed to the valley, and life has resumed its comforting rhythms.

* * * *

Saw the doctor this morning. The report is not good. My tumors have grown under this new treatment so we are going to have to go back on chemo. After going through all of the various options (and we talked about six or seven) we decided that I will try Xeloda and Herceptin. I should not lose my hair this time, although I will feel fatigue. I hope it isn't like the last chemo when I could barely walk across the street without stopping three times. I may also get mouth sores, diarrhea, or hand and foot syndrome. So we discussed what I need to look for.

I have to get an echocardiogram at the end of this week to get a baseline since the Herceptin can cause heart damage and needs to be managed. Then I see the doc again next Tuesday. If the echo is OK and the insurance is OK then I might get my first Herceptin treatment on that visit. The schedule is that I will have intravenous Herceptin weekly for three weeks and then once every three weeks thereafter. The Xeloda is in pill form so I will have to take four pills each morning and evening for two weeks and then take one week off and start again.

I was thinking as I was leaving the doctor's office that if I have to fight this disease, how much more pleasant it is to fight it here in Kalispell rather than in a large city. The hospital is 5 minutes (not 30 minutes) from the house, I don't have to pay for parking (vs. $15 each visit), and scheduling procedures is a snap (vs. having to wait for a week or two). It is just easier and my oncologist is a brilliant doctor who really knows her medicine and knows her patients; so much better than my first oncologist in D.C. So rather than mull over this as a cruel twist of fate that as soon as I got here this happened, I am thankful that if it was going to happen, that I am here. Life is still wonderful and abundant!

My friends and I are taking a three-day float trip in a month to fish the southern part of the Flathead River. It will be a wonderful time through outrageously gorgeous scenery. We will eat great Dutch oven dinners and catch lots of fish and laugh and talk trash. It doesn't get any better than this. And if I am too fatigued to fish, I'll just sit in the boat and look and listen and still have a great time. I'll keep you posted as I go through the next phase of this adventure.

* * * *

In clinical terms I seem to be an outlier; every cytotoxin I have ever been on has tried to kill me. This time it was the Xeloda. After ten days of being on treatment I ended up in the hospital with every single side effect listed and then some. My gastrointestinal tract is burned and blistered from mouth to bottom. I had hand/foot syndrome, an infection they could never identify but that Cipro knocked out, massive explosive diarrhea and subsequent dehydration, phenomenal gut pain, and a fungal infection on my skin. I was also anemic and my ketones and liver function tests were off the charts.

I was in the hospital for seven days before they would trust me to come home. Eating has been a torture but I have worked my way up from fats and meats to whole grain. Once I master that I get to move on to cooked veggies. Yahoo! The upshot of all of this is that I have decided that I will not do traditional chemo anymore. I will continue on with Herceptin and treatments like Avastin, but the traditional cytotoxins I will steer clear of.

This has been a decision that has been hard on my friends and family. We are so bought into the scientific studies of treatment outcomes that we forget that the science really only works on a bell curve. If you have someone like me who does not fit within the bell, you really don't know what the treatment is going to do.

I am convinced now that if I do traditional treatment, it will not just make me miserable, it will kill me. So I have decided to take my chances on feeling better for whatever time I have left. It may be short or long, but at least I won't be in the hospital wishing I was dead already. Bill supports me in this although it has raised a lot of emotions for him that I think he would prefer not to deal with. We won't know what this decision means in terms of longevity until I have my next scans. That may not be for three months so we are living in limbo to some extent, but we are indeed living each moment and that is the point.

* * * *

Update: I feel terrific! I have gotten over the results of the last treatment. The only problems now are that chemo over time has messed with my mind so that I have an attention deficit problem. We have recently discovered that this is the reason that I have been falling so frequently. I have no balance problem when I'm not distracted, but if I try to do the same exercises and hold a conversation at the same time I am likely to fall down. Oh well, so I need to learn how to focus again. My next scans are the third week of July. That is when we find out if this Herceptin program is effective. I will keep you posted as soon as I know something.

* * * *

Dear friends! It has been so long since I have checked in with you. I am happy to report that I am feeling better than I have in the past two years. I started a new medicine, Tykerb, about three months ago, in conjunction with the Herceptin. It takes awhile for any effects of this type of treatment to be felt so it hasn't been until recently that I have been able to report a major change. I am not coughing as much, am not tired, and do not experience nearly the amount of pain I have in the past. Yahoo! And to testify to this salutary effect, I have just returned from a rigorous three-week trip to Scotland, where I toured Glasgow, the Trossachs and the Hebrides with another friend, on our own, and using public transportation.

The trip was remarkable not only for what I did and saw, and for being with a number of dear friends I haven't seen for awhile, but for the change in my emotional outlook. I am now thinking more about living than about dying. I had a brain MRI this past week to see if I have any brain mets. I will get the results tomorrow, but I do not expect anything to show up. I have been having horrible headaches, but they went away when I got to Scotland so I believe they are allergy related. In any case we will see.

Thank all of you for your prayers and positive wishes and thoughts. This is a long roller-coaster ride of a disease and it takes a lot to continue caring over such a long time. Your prayers have a lot to do with the fact the meds seem to be working and I cannot thank you enough.

On another positive note, the chemotherapy drug that I am waiting for has been sent to the FDA for approval. I don't know how long it will take. It had been fast-tracked for approval but then they started seeing problems with Avastin, another cancer drug they had fast-tracked, so everything is now off the fast track and it will get approved whenever it gets approved. I will continue to keep you posted as things unfold. Many thanks and much love!

* * * *

Quick update. Had scans yesterday of my lung mets. My oncologist just called me because she thought I would like to hear that my "tumors are shrinking nicely!" Yahoo. It's the first time that they have shrunk rather than growing or just staying the same size.

* * * *

Since the last time I wrote I have been on a new treatment that shrank the tumors and then that treatment failed. I go to the oncologist tomorrow to see where we go from here. In the meantime, this wonderful article in *The Times* appeared that does an excellent job of describing how metastatic breast cancer is very different from non-Stage IV cancer. Here is the link for those of you who seek to understand more about my experience. "A Pink-Ribbon Race, Years Long" by Roni Caryn Rabin, published January 17, 2011: http://www.nytimes.com/2011/01/18/health/18cancer.html?pagewanted=all.

I also am happy to report that in spite of this new setback I have outlasted the average life expectancy with this diagnosis by two months!

* * * *

I am sitting in the chemo room waiting for my infusion, having just met with my onc. At this point we are not changing anything pending a conference with a surgical oncologist. I raised the issue that there is really one problematic tumor that doesn't pay any attention and keeps growing. Is it possible to treat that one tumor locally? While it will require thinking a bit outside the box of normal therapy, my doc thinks it is at least worth looking into.

She has scheduled me for a visit with a surgical oncologist, not specifically for a surgical solution, but to at least be evaluated for the possibility of different therapies like ablation and radioseeds. If it works, this won't cure the cancer but it will give me a bit more time before I have to go back on a harsh chemo. The surgeon may not be able to do anything but it is worth a shot. I also have been concerned that chemo may ruin my summer plans.

While this sounds silly to most of you, we live through a long dark winter for the pleasure of the eight weeks of summer. I missed summer last year because of hospitalization and rehabilitation; I am not missing this summer and the fabulous float trips we have already planned. Gotta get on the river. My doc assured me that she will work around these plans so I can go. I will report in again once we know in which direction we are headed. I am feeling a bit less scared for now.

* * * *

Just a short update. I saw the surgical oncologist yesterday and after a long conversation about philosophies of treatment he agreed to go in and get the visible tumors using radio frequency ablation. This is most likely not going to be a cure (I wasn't asking for one) but it will reset the clock a bit and we will be able to look at the metabolic profile of the maverick tumor that grows regardless of what we throw at it, and that looks very different on the scans than the other tumors.

So I am scheduled for surgery on my left lung May 11. We will then see how I do and if I'm OK we will schedule the right lung by early June. The only reason that we are able to do this is because the tumors have not spread to other organs. In this I am much more fortunate than most other women going through this. Pure grace! I'm very grateful. Good story for Easter about the power of the Resurrection. I will keep you updated on the saga.

* * * *

Hi all! Just to bring you up to date. I had my first lung surgery a month ago. They ablated a tumor in the upper lobe of my right lung and excised a huge one in the lower lobe. The immediate results were that I stopped coughing and I now have color in my face, even roses in my cheeks, for the first time in over three years. It is so exciting! The only negative from it is that I have tremendous unremitting nerve pain on my lower rib. The doc says this is because they had to put in a drain there as well as it being in the way of the excision. I have not been given a pain killer for nerve pain, and the traditional oxycodone doesn't do anything for it. Today was the worst. Having to breathe in short shallow breaths. Will talk to the doc again on Monday about changing medications. This should be temporary but in some cases it becomes chronic. Crossed fingers.

My second surgery is scheduled for this coming Wednesday, June 8. It will be far more invasive and they will have to spread my ribs for it. I will be in the hospital close to six days for this one. I have a huge gnarly looking tumor in the upper lobe which will necessitate a lobectomy. The surgeon is going to try and save a portion of the upper lobe but might have to take it all to get it out. Then there is another tumor in the lower lobe which will be more straightforward and less of a challenge. The plan is that after this surgery I will be NED (no evidence of disease) for the first time in three years. We do not know how long I will be in this state; it may be for a few weeks or it may be longer. In any case it will be wonderful to have at least reset the cancer clock a bit. I cannot believe how much more energy I have just from having the right lung cleared. Bill better watch out because I may be pumped up, LOL!

This is truly the miracle we have been praying for. A surgical solution is rarely employed in cases of Stage 4 breast cancer. Unlike other cancers, breast cancer likes to seed itself throughout the body and pop up now and again. My situation is very unusual in that my tumors are only in my lungs and not in liver and bones or brain. The fact that I don't have new tumors, but only the same ones we have been dealing with since the beginning, gives the doctors hope that I will be one of the few where a surgical solution may be exactly that, a solution, and that the cancer may be gone after this. I am not counting on it but it is a possibility. My doctors have used surgery to deal with a breast cancer metastasis only once before (even though they have been physicians for a long time) and I am the second case so clearly they are hopeful that this will have positive results. They are all very excited for me and about this case so I hope that I am able to provide that bright spot that they don't often see with Stage 4 breast cancer.

Thanks for your prayers and support. They have brought us to this point. I am very excited although not looking forward to the recovery, but I have a beautiful and comfortable home, a wonderful caring husband, loads of wonderful loyal friends, and downloadable ebooks. What else could a girl want! I will write again once I am through the recovery and back on my feet. Blessings!

* * * *

I have had a number of people e-mailing me with concern as they haven't heard from me since the second surgery. I apologize. The surgery was a success! I was in the hospital for ten days. I am still in a lot of pain and learning how to breathe with my reduced lung capacity. Get fatigued extraordinarily easily. All of this will resolve but will take time. Bill is doing a wonderful job of caring for me. I will write more later when it isn't so taxing. Lots of love to you all!

* * * *

Hi friends. Well, as I promised, I am reporting in after my first post-op scans. The results were mixed, as I have come to expect. On the positive side: often after surgery, like the type I had, cancer tumors begin to sprout like a mushroom farm. There is something in the process of healing that also spurs tumor growth. This did not happen, so I am very grateful and take that as a sign that my disease is not widespread. On the negative side, they did find another nodule that might be a new tumor. But just one. It is small and located near an incision line. We cannot biopsy it nor can we take it out surgically due to its location near the scarring. Thus, we can only wait and see.

Given that I am taking two drugs that retard the explosive

growth that my cancer is capable of, we feel confident that, if it is cancerous, it will grow at a slow enough rate to give us time to respond. There are still some post-op issues that will resolve over time and I am feeling pretty good. Have spent a lot of time on the river this summer and vastly improved my fly casting. Learning to enjoy each day without regard to accomplishment; a big deal for me! Until next time.

* * * *

Saw oncologist today to get results of latest CT scan. Unfortunately the tumor is growing again. We are not sure what we are going to do next in terms of treatment. Unless I agree to go back on cytotoxic chemo there are few, if any, other options for me. So, oncologist is going to track down some information on one newly approved. I do not qualify for any clinical trials given my weird disease. I am going to check out information on the vitamin C infusions and we are to meet again next week to decide what, if anything, to do differently.

* * * *

So much has happened since I last wrote. It has been the typical roller-coaster ride; one minute you're up and then you're down. I went to see the surgical oncologist for another opinion on the recent growth. He saw the nodule that they found as a failure on his part to take a large enough margin when he excised the tumor and felt that it could, in fact, be dealt with surgically on an outpatient basis through interventional radiology.

I then learned from the surgical oncologist that they had biopsied six lymph nodes around my heart and when the surgery biopsy results came back all six were found to be cancerous. So, not knowing about the six nodes, thinking that there was only one tumor that could easily be dealt with had initially gotten my hopes up. But, given the six nodes and before submitting to another procedure on my poor beleaguered body, I went for a PET scan to see if there might be disease elsewhere. No point in taking out a tumor if there is another one left behind.

The PET scan was not as favorable as I had wished. It showed that, in addition to the nodule, I had cancer in two lymph nodes and possibly at two sites in my spine and ribs. So instead of being happy about getting rid of the nodule I now had to realize that I had more systemic disease and start thinking about drugs again.

It is so hard when you are given two choices and they both have such horrible potential side effects. You really do have to pick your poison. One option would have given me neuropathy which is the worst for me. I need to be able to feel my feet if I am to ski or to wade in a stream fishing.

So, even though it had good statistical data on its efficacy, I decided on the other option. I am now on treatment protocol that involves an off-label use of Afinitor in conjunction with Aromasin. While the FDA has not approved this usage, the data on this protocol is quite strong and shows benefit even for women with triple negative breast cancer (now, the hardest to treat). It will be another two to three months before I have a CT to show what is happening.

I have now been on it 13 days and the side effects, so far, have been manageable. I am fatigued and having occasional nose bleeds. I am told by two other women I know who just started this same protocol a few weeks before I did that I also have to look forward to an unpleasant taste in my mouth that will make food unpalatable. That may not be altogether bad; since I had the lung surgery I have gained over twenty pounds and now look like a well-tended 4-H pig at the state fair. There are also lots of impact on blood levels so we will see when I have my next blood draw on Wednesday. It is supposed to increase blood sugar and cholesterol.

On the positive side, the FDA has committed to release its

decision on pertuzumab on June 8. Pertuzumab has had strong clinical trials and is a drug that I should benefit from. So I am keeping crossed fingers for if this is approved it will be the next drug in my arsenal. (I have used up all the options that don't cause neuropathy.) TDM-1, which is a super charged version of Herceptin, will conclude its clinical trials this year and they will apply to the FDA by the end of the year for marketing approval. It is another drug that has had excellent results in trials that would benefit me. I suspect it will be two years before it will be available on the market if at all.

My oncologist's office now has a naturopath on staff part-time and they are beginning to use her to help ameliorate side effects. I have been lobbying for intravenous vitamin C, which has shown tremendous benefit in easing side effects of chemo in trials, and the office is now in a position to offer that at last. They also finally have a clinical social worker available to oncology outpatients. I have met with her and she was very helpful and will be a good resource for me when needed. Sad to say, she is the only social worker at the hospital who does counseling as the rest are relegated to discharge planning. The hospital is committed to being a designated cancer center and will be building a new facility starting next year which will house all oncology resources under one roof. I will let you know how this treatment goes. From what I understand the side effects build for about a month and then level off. I sure hope it works!

* * * *

Thank all of you so much for the continuing prayer support. This disease is so taxing on all of us and I am grateful for your steadfast support over this long, and hopefully long-er, haul. First an update: I have now been on my new treatment regimen for a month and am tolerating it fairly well. The primary side effect that impacts my quality of life is overwhelming fatigue, but we have been able to reschedule our anniversary trip out another six months so I have time now to adjust to the treatment with no pressure. It is an amazing drug and I am very hopeful, even though I am bummed about not being able to do things right now.

I have two prayer requests which may seem somewhat silly but are not. The most emergent one is that we need to find a housekeeper because our experience with the maid services here is that they are expensive and do not do a very good job. I am at a loss as to how to find someone good who will take a personal interest in our well-being and how she/he could contribute to it (and that we can afford). Bill is doing as much as he can but he is not well either and while he is doing the marketing and most of the cooking, cleaning is too physically demanding on him. My treatment suppresses my immune system and so a clean house is really critical for me.

Secondly is a prayer for the FDA. They are to rule on the first new drug out of the pipeline for quite some time in early June, pertuzumab, and we are hopeful that they will approve it. The prayer request, however, is for a different drug – TDM-1 which is the first of the biologics to marry a cytotoxin with a biologic. The biologic will be attracted to the most rapidly dividing cells and will then deliver the cytotoxin only to those cells and not to the whole body. The approval got tied up in politics last year regarding another drug approval so they have been taking their time on this. I covet your prayers that the FDA consider this and render a decision quickly. There are so many of us that are waiting on this drug as our last chance. I am not there yet but if the treatment I am on now is not effective I will be in that category.

* * * *

Just a short update. We have found a housekeeper and I am

thrilled. She was suggested to me by a mutual friend. So, I think I can relax now and know that we will be able to manage with this help. The fatigue from this new treatment continues to be a problem. I did some preparatory cleaning yesterday (you know we all clean before the cleaner comes) and am paying for it big time today. But, it was nice to have been active even though I did have to rest in between. Now I know that I can achieve some level of activity every once in awhile as long as I plan out recuperation time on the back end. I see the oncologist this week as well as have my every-three-weeks infusion of Herceptin so I know I will be sick for a few days afterwards. I am taking three different cancer drugs that work on three different mechanisms and the Herceptin infusions just seem to break my back every time. Just one medicine too many for my body, but the reaction is short-lived fortunately.

* * * *

I have been asked to write something since it has been a long time since I have written. This is the chronic part of this disease, it is long periods of boredom interspersed with moments of terror. Right now things are fairly stable. My last CT was a little funky and we don't know exactly what it means so we will have to wait another three months before we find out. I have one tumor in my lung and I have cancer in a number of lymph nodes surrounding my heart. The last scan shows even more swollen nodes. Is it cancer or is it sarcoidosis or something else? No idea. My insurance company has notified me that it will no longer pay for one of the three cancer medications that I am currently taking. Our appeal has been denied. We have petitioned the drug company for relief on the price and are waiting for their response. At over $4,000 per month (for only that one drug) there is no way we can pay for it out of pocket. It is not working that well, but at least it is slowing the cancer down so to lose it before something comes along to replace it in my regimen is serious.

This treatment regimen that I am currently on is the last available one for me. If the FDA does not approve some new drugs I will be out of luck when this regimen completely fails, probably within the next few months. But on the positive side, a new drug is scheduled to be ruled on by the FDA by the end of Feb. if not before. The drug trials have been highly successful and my doctor and I have our fingers crossed that it will be available for me. So just have to wait and see. Meanwhile, after having a low red blood count for a number of months due to chemo, this month the count nearly fell off the chart so I was pleased to get a blood transfusion yesterday and feel quite a bit better. One of the side effects of my current treatment is hemorrhaging and we are running some tests to see if the recent low counts were due to internal bleeding of some sort.

* * * *

The hardest part of my situation is having friends diagnosed with the same condition or friends with other cancers who receive difficult news. Trying to be positive in the face of this at times is difficult. I continue to look well, though a little heavy again due to medications. This bothers some people who, I guess, feel that I am only worthy of their concern if I am gaunt and feeble. They don't understand how important it is for me to feel normal and to look normal and I spend time trying to put on the best face possible. This is a marathon not a sprint and I can't bear feeling the weight of this disease and others' expectations over the amount of time it will take to play out. I think I have adjusted to my new normal, but every time I think that the disease throws a new challenge at me. Life is still delicious and I enjoy a reasonable quality of life. I will write again when I have news or if too much boring time has gone by so you will know I am OK.

* * * *

Just was called by my oncologist and test results show I am bleeding internally, we just don't know where. So more procedures to follow to try and figure out what is happening and I get to add another doctor to my cadre! I told my doctor that I didn't want her to be bored and to consider this her Christmas present! She is wonderful and I am grateful for her care.

* * * *

Dear friends, I have been so excited about the new drug that has just been approved by the FDA, Kadcyla. It is the first smart bomb drug for breast cancer and I was looking forward to going on it when my current prescription runs out. You see, the insurance company has refused to pay for the drug I am currently on so I will be forced to change treatments in three weeks. I wasn't worried because I thought that I could go on Kadcyla. Unfortunately, when I looked at the new Kadcyla Web site it states that Kadcyla is only available to women with metastatic breast cancer who have failed treatment with both Herceptin and a taxane.

For the four years we have been fighting this cancer we have avoided the taxanes because they can cause nerve damage and neuropathy. I had polio as a child and I already am suffering from damaged nerves and we did not want to make things worse. So, we are going to have to petition my insurance company for a waiver for them to agree to pay for the new cancer medication. Although taxanes shrink tumors, they also cause permanent nerve damage and release so many live cancer cells into the bloodstream that it is questionable whether they actually prolong life. Nevertheless, regardless of these negatives, they are included in almost all breast cancer treatment regimens on the fact that they do shrink tumors.

Unfortunately I am currently on my ninth treatment protocol and, other than the taxanes or Kadcyla, there are no options left for me. So I am seemingly between the devil and the deep blue sea if the insurance company will not pay for Kadcyla. I can either go on the taxanes and lose the feeling in my feet and hands, or I can die. Those are my two choices. Sucks to be me. So please pray that the insurance company will agree to pay for the new drug for me so that I can avoid the taxanes. It is really a matter of life or death. Thanks!

* * * *

Since I last wrote I have gotten the results of my last CT scan. Two of my tumors actually had areas of necrosis for the first time in four and a half years! So it seems this treatment protocol that I am on (yes, the one the insurance company has refused to pay for) is working. I saw my oncologist today after having a telephone conference with her last week. She searched around her office and came up with enough of this medication to keep me going for the next 90 days. I am due another CT in 90 days and we will see then how we proceed. It may be possible, if those results also show the tumors are dying, to have the insurance company revisit its decision. In any case, we are not going to try to make the change to Kadcyla quite yet. I am hoping that either there will be more drugs turned in and samples to keep me going, or that the results will present a compelling case. Thank you all for your prayers.

I am out of strength right now. It just gets better and better (sarcasm) than I imagined. You get so frightened when you are in this situation that you cannot see straight and that is why your prayers are so vital to keeping me from falling apart. So we will keep on the current path and I will not have to adjust to a new medication. It's as good a result as one could ask for.

* * * *

I am now finding myself between the proverbial rock and hard place. I have scans tomorrow and then meet with my oncologist next week to decide on treatment. I suspect that the existing treatment is no longer working, at least the side effects are pretty gnarly and may not be tolerable for much longer. That being said I have gotten a year out of it, which, as cancer goes, is pretty good.

My wonderful new drug, Kadcyla, for which I have prayed is now available but there is a hitch. My insurer will not pay for it unless I have first been on a taxane. The problem is that taxanes cause nerve damage, and as someone with a history of polio and existing nerve damage, it could and probably will make the nerve damage worse. So my choices boil down to this: take the taxanes (jump through that hoop for the insurance company) and risk permanent nerve damage and possible loss of my legs, or don't do anything and die. Pretty easy choice right?

I am tired and demoralized. I am tired of seeing my cancer friends die. I am overwhelmed with my husband's Parkinson's and with life in general. I don't know what I am going to do but I will say that I am flirting with dying. I have never been at this point before and it scares me but I may really be ready to just let go. It is all beginning to seem pointless. So… prayers coveted to get through this.

* * * *

OK, friends, I just got the call from my oncologist with the results of my scans. As usual they were a mixed bag: some tumors shrank and some grew. But the kicker is that I now have heart failure caused by the cancer drugs. Doc is extremely concerned to the point that treating my heart failure now trumps my cancer so I will be taken off cancer drugs for a bit until we can get the heart in better shape. Crap!

It is so funny because you go along and feel relatively OK and you forget that cancer is, after all, the big C cancer until this happens and now I remember that I am really sick! Anyway, I hope to see a cardiologist sometime this week and then go from there. So we still don't know what we are going to do about the taxanes (to taxane or not to taxane, that is the question). But we do know that this heart failure has to be treated now. No wonder my feet and ankles were so swollen on our trip!

* * * *

Met with oncologist today to map out possible next steps, post-cardiac stabilization. All new chemos cause neuropathy and most taxanes require steroids. Between having had polio and being allergic to steroids there isn't much choice. Given my physical meltdown with cytotoxins, oncologist believes that I lack the enzyme to metabolize them so we will have to proceed very cautiously. See her again in one month. Now it's time to see cardiologist and see if heart is stabilizing.

* * * *

Love, love, love my cardiologist! One of the best patient communicators I have ever seen. Have a full understanding of what is going on, what we are facing, and what we have to do to get through this. Start medications tonight. She says I will feel like crap for the next week and then I will feel better in time for them to adjust the medications and make me feel like crap again. Hmmm, sounds like chemo. I can do this! CT in ten days to peek at what the cancer is doing in the meantime. Will keep you posted.

* * * *

I had a CT scan last week to see how the disease is progressing now that we have taken me off Herceptin. Herceptin is a great drug for HER2 positive breast cancer, which is the most aggressive form. We were concerned that the loss of it would mean that the cancer would take off like a rocket but, for whatever reason, that has not happened. The scans show that my tumors are stable. So, because of this great news we have put off the switch to the taxane a bit longer.

I am still on two other cancer medications that seem to be holding the fort so we will continue with them until they no longer work. My heart is responding to treatment as well and I am feeling better than I have in a couple of years! Even talking about rejoining the health club and working out. We are still titrating the medicines so not at a stable place yet but I am very encouraged. I see the cardiologist in two more weeks. This is such a roller-coaster experience; one minute sheer terror and the next a bit of bliss. Thanks for hanging in with me.

* * * *

Since August things have been a bit hairy here. I have been dropping weight and can see a new tumor growing out of my neck. I have never been able to see my tumors before and it is a little freaky. I have lost my ability to speak due to tumors pressing up against my larynx and feel like someone is choking me most of the time. I am so short of breath and fatigued that I now am walking with a walker to help conserve energy. We have been holding back on treating the cancer until my heart was functioning normally again. I can now say, with great thanksgiving, that my heart is pumping at normal levels.

* * * *

I missed my chemo today because I was seeing a radiation oncologist, and an ENT, and scheduling surgery for Monday. It seems my vocal chords are paralyzed and my diaphragm might be as well. It is life threatening so I have opted to have a tracheostomy so that I can breathe more easily. The problem was caused by tumors interfering with the nerves that control these. I opted not to have radiation now because it might cause swelling in an already tight space, plus I get to save it in case things get hairy later. I will have my first chemo tomorrow. I will be in the hospital for a few days after the surgery. Not looking forward to any of this but glad we have an answer.

* * * *

I was scheduled to go in for surgery on Monday to have the trach put in. Friday night I felt so awful that I woke up Saturday and a voice in my head stated unequivocally, "This is really stupid... you need to go to the hospital now."

So I woke up Bill and said he needed to take me to the hospital now! He called the ENT's office and made arrangements and we went off to the emergency room. I already knew that I was scheduled for Monday, but the ER docs began their own further examination of me. I had CT scans and chest x-rays, I had so many blood tests I began to look pale. More and more doctors jumped on board.

Eventually we all got drawn into the dancing of the dizzy on-call cardiologists as new tests resurrected that old bugaboo the tamponade, the ridiculous discussion of which, "No, she has too much other stuff going on so it couldn't possibly be a tamponade," you have been spared. It was indeed a tamponade along with everything else. There was more liquid surrounding my heart and it now was impacting my heart's ability to beat. So the one thing they could agree on was that it was not going to get any better. So, finally, I needed a cardiac window cut into the wall of the cardiac sac in order for the water to drain out and keep the heart from being compromised.

Both of these were considered life threatening so there was no question of me going home. I was admitted on Saturday afternoon. Monday morning I had both surgeries and they were hard, but the tracheotomy was the worst, even more so than the lung surgery I had earlier. It was the worst because of the overwhelming belief that you were going to suffocate to death. I couldn't speak, breathe, control my voice. It was a totally different me that was peeking out of my eyes and trying to communicate, mostly through grotesque facial gestures and monosyllabic answers.

The first trach was switched out for a smaller and lighter one that I could breathe with and make some modicum of intelligible sound. But eating was and still is a nightmare. Every swallow ends in choking and coughing and problem solving of how to handle this. Every cough sounds like a weed-whacker starting up on a Saturday morning before 6:00am. It is jarring and scares little children.

I have finally been discharged with a boatload of equipment to be dealt with. I will have home health nurses coming to check on me. When I started this I had thought that I would be able to fix these problems and end up my old self. The lessons of this past week say that that is not going to happen. I am now instantly old with a trach and a walker and a creeping walk. It is to be seen whether continuing on with this fight was brave or an ill-conceived thought of cowardice.

* * * *

A friend of mine has a nickname for cancer, whack-a-mole. It is so true. Whenever you think you have it dialed in something unexpected comes at you from left field, you are knocked off your balance and have to adjust. It happens quickly and is disorienting.

I have had a few of those moments in the past two months. Firstly, my quality of life was terrible and I was physically really suffering. My work with a palliative doctor was just starting and not having much effect. I was not sure I wanted to keep living if this is what life would be like 'til the end. I lost more weight and could not get enough nutrients. To add insult to injury I also fell on the ice ten days ago and broke my right wrist.

The palliative doc said she was worried and that if I couldn't counter the rapid weight loss she was afraid that I wouldn't be alive much longer. We were tasked quite sternly to go home and tie up any unfinished business because when the time came it would be fast. Whoa!

Bill and I went home and reevaluated how we might get me to eat again. Food was not enticing at all, and even though we had focused on calorie loading, I was still only offered food at normal meal times. We decided to feed me tiny portions every two hours. Slowly I began to eat more during the course of a day. My gastrointestinal tract started working properly again and after about eight to ten days I began to be hungry. Even though I am still eating calorie-laden foods my weight is stable and not gaining, but you have to start somewhere.

So two weeks after this wake-up call and food campaign commenced, it was time for my quarterly CT to see what the cancer was doing. I did not know what to expect with the whole death knell thing hanging over my head, but I expected they would be good as I could actually see the tumors shrinking. So here is the whipsaw, after having been told two weeks earlier that there was a very real chance I could die soon, the CT came back with the amazing news that my cancer was in remission! They saw nothing!

Whoa! Talk about whiplash. I will take it. My heart failure is completely reversed and my cancer is not measurable. With less tumor burden I now am beginning to have more energy, and it is wonderful to look in the mirror and see fat pink cheeks instead of the gaunt gray ones I have had for so long.

We do not know how long this will last, it could be only weeks or it could extend out years. We need to be in a place where we can be comfortable in the not knowing. Meanwhile, for people in my condition, treatment doesn't stop just because the cancer is in remission. I will stay on this chemo for another five to six weeks and then we will reconsider what maintenance drug changes should be made.

First of all, miracles do happen and those of you who have been on this journey with me since the beginning know that I have experienced many miracles and last minute saves over this course. Thank you for the prayers and support because you have had a hand in bringing this about.

The second thing, which I need to process before saying too much about, is that there is a huge spiritual component in this new status. Some of you know that I have been working with a shaman over the past eighteen months because I felt that the tenacity of my otherwise well-behaved cancer must have a spiritual nexus. I continue to be convinced of this fact and have work to be done yet. How it will ultimately play out with the cancer I do not know but deep things are rocking my world and it is very interesting to be me right now!

* * * *

Back in the hospital. Problem is gastroparesis… impacts ability to both eat and digest. In phenomenal pain.

It is serious and may impact my survival.

Not up for more talk. Bill or I will update when crisis is past.

* * * *

This has been a tough week but on the other hand they now know what has been plaguing me for months now. After I took myself to the ER again, they did their usual stellar job and found that my stomach is paralyzed and essentially does nothing. It has been doing nothing for some time, not even emptying, so it is very distended. My surgeon wants to enter me in the Nathan's Hotdog contest and is sure we would win!

The scary thing is that there is a phenomenon with some cancer patients where cancerous lymph nodes in the chest area surrounding the esophagus slowly squeeze off the vagus nerve resulting in the paralysis of the entire GI track. Since my vocal chords and stomach are both paralyzed they are concerned that this might be happening to me. If it does that is the end.

For now my intestines are working well and so tomorrow they are putting in a feeding tube. It will bypass my esophagus (which is trashed and bleeding) and stomach and deliver nutrition directly to my small bowel where I can digest it. This nutrition is specially for situations like this and will be delivered by a machine through a tube attached to a port on my belly. Because my stomach will not empty I cannot eat very much at all. I am hopeful that I can from time to time have something yummy but probably not more than once a month.

My esophagus is "raw meat" according to the gastroenterologist. As a result I have been bleeding and losing iron. After I was discharged from the hospital on Thursday I was readmitted on Friday (ambulance ride and much drama) because I had lost so many red blood cells that it was life threatening. During the course of the weekend I was given two units of packed cells and an iron transfusion to try and jump-start my bone marrow to make more red blood cells. This was successful and I left feeling better than I have in ages.

So, I don't know what is ahead. This is the best decision I can make with the information at my disposal. I cannot forecast the future, only just live today. Having adequate nutrition is going to be something new for me and I am looking forward to feeling better.

* * * *

The oddest thing happened. I was in the endoscopy suite, prepped for the surgery and anesthetized. Because my stomach is so stretched and distended, when the doc went to place the valve for the tube, he could not use the spot he needed as it was tucked behind a rib. So the operation was aborted. Later the doc said that he wanted to see me in another week and we would decide how to proceed. He also said that my stomach did seem to be doing a little something and he wanted to see if that continued.

On the one hand I was really glad not to have another hole carved into me, but on the other hand eating has been a horror and I was looking forward to the assurance that the feedings would provide adequate nutrition and calories. In the three days since the surgery snafu, even eating every two hours, I have lost another five pounds.

Bill checked in with him today and he seems to think things are going fine. We are to call him next Tuesday. I may need to get the other big guns to pitch in so that I am convinced my best interests are being looked after.

Well, time to eat again! Details will be provided as they are available.

* * * *

This is the second week after the surgery was supposed to take place but the docs have again asked me to try and eat on my own for another week and then we will revisit whether to do the surgery.

On the positive side, I have gotten more familiar with foods that will leave the stomach quickly and it has gotten easier to eat every two hours and still not have any discomfort. The question remains: is the amount I am able to eat going to be enough to maintain my weight? We will see. The first week after the surgery date I lost another six pounds. This week, it is not clear at this point, but don't think I am losing as quickly. If I can maintain my weight the docs will be very pleased and there will be no surgery. If I cannot we will have to revisit it again from all angles.

* * * *

A friend has asked me to update the site since I haven't written in a while. There really isn't much to tell. I have been able to maintain my weight finally without the surgery. We are getting better at preparing meals I can eat although the amount of meat and the frequency I can eat it are still problematic. Bill made some killer enchiladas suisas for me that tasted wonderful and didn't tax my system.

The emotional toll of the past few months has been heavy, and I am only now coming out of the doldrums. I learned today that someone I know had a medical crisis that has left him a quadriplegic and, when I contemplate what that must be like, things on my end do not seem quite so dire.

The trach continues to be a thorn as I have coughing spasms and times when I can't clear my throat and end up making this very loud and rude noise in the process. There is no way I can maintain a facade of normalcy in public. People are either weirded out when they see me or they treat me as though I were a child or feeble elder. I now speak with a piping lilt that has the same effect on telephone calls. I am sick of teenage sales clerks calling me "dear."

The crise de jour is neuropathy. The chemo I have just completed has left me with numb and tingling hands and feet. As we had feared, it has also attacked my polio-damaged legs and I cannot walk any longer without assistance. I am thankful for my rollator because it helps me remain standing and gives me a way to sit when my legs have had enough. I have also learned that numb fingers mean difficulties getting dressed, writing, or even holding on to something. We are hopeful that the neuropathy will fade over time but there is no guarantee.

I am now on a chemo holiday of unknown duration. In a month we will have another CT and see if the cancer has reappeared. If it hasn't, the holiday may be extended. If it has, then I will move on to a new chemotherapy. This will be the course for the rest of my life.

It is hard to be upbeat because my quality of life sucks. It is all well and good if I thought a meaningful life was one where I stay curled on the couch watching movies on my computer, but that is not me, although that has been my life for the past three months. Bill continues to tell me that it is important to him that I am still around, so for him I take a deep breath and hold on. But, I can't hike, fish, ski, or even hold my pistol so I could go to the range for some diversion. I can still see the mountains outside my window and that is a source of peace for me. I have the consolation of being where I most want to be in the world.

Sorry I am not all happy and a paragon of well-being but I set out to be truthful about this experience and the road is just getting rockier. It is hard and not pleasant and will not end well. Perhaps when spring arrives things will seem better. I do have excellent friends here who do lovely things to give me a lift; this would be intolerable otherwise.

I thank you for your continued love and prayers. They mean the world, especially right now.

* * * *

I have just come from the oncologist where I got the results of the recent CT scan. The cancer is back primarily in the mediastinal lymph nodes, the ones that paralyzed my vocal chords and stomach. I will be starting a new chemotherapy drug as soon as the insurance company has approved it.

The drug I will be on, God willing, is Kadcyla. It is the smart bomb drug TDM-1. The results of the clinical studies showed that it substantially lengthened the time until progression and had fewer side effects. I prayed for this drug to be approved for three years and now will be able to take it.

There may be some cardiotoxic effects but I just had an echocardiogram that showed my heart is stable and functioning well once again. I hope it stays that way while I am on this drug because there are no other alternatives.

It looks like chemotherapy will be a constant until I die. Bill and I are taking stock and trying to decide if there are things we ought to do now because it is fairly certain I won't be able to do them in the fairly near future.

Spring has arrived and with it a rebirth, not of hope for the future necessarily, but of a sense of the possible. I have been able to take very short walks outside which have boosted my spirits. Bill has assured me that we will get through this and I choose to believe him.

* * * *

I have been on Kadcyla for four infusions now. It is very kind to my noncancerous cells and I am feeling better than I have in quite a while. I actually was able to do a very short hike a couple of weeks ago for the first time in over two years. I had scans last week and the chemotherapy is working well. Next scans in October. As they say: scan, treat, repeat. That's my life. I will update when I have more news.

* * * *

Well friends, just as I was trying to figure out living my next stage, having gotten used to the trach and managing reasonably well with the frozen stomach, something else has arisen which needs to be checked out. I have had a difficult couple of days and yesterday was very difficult. I have seen my oncologist and we are worried the cancer has spread to my brain. So we have scheduled an MRI for next Thursday with results following Monday. So far today I am reasonably OK; not as much difficulty walking or standing and the room isn't spinning, etc. But very very tired. Trying not to jump to conclusions but the fear is always just below the surface.

Nevertheless, I am not letting this take away from my delight in life, or at least not to a great extent. We are still planning on having a dear friend come stay with us next month and on taking another mini-vacation to the Salish Lodge in Snoqualmie, WA in early Oct. If I can locomote and can wake up a bit better tomorrow there is a bear symposium sponsored by Vital Ground that I want to attend as well as a concert by the Drum Brothers tomorrow night in Bigfork. But, as it will be a rainy and cool weekend, it is always good for a book and a movie.

I covet your prayers that the tests will give the docs some idea of what has been happening to me. I also pray it is not cancer in my brain. My brain is such a huge part of my self-identity and my enjoyment of life that losing even a small amount of function is very hard to contemplate.

For those of you who know I have been having bone pain in my spine, the brain issue trumps the bones for now. Given the last CT report, the oncologist does not think that the malformation seen by the radiologist in my spine is cancer. If the pain persists we will do a PET scan but for now we have much bigger fish to fry!!

* * * *

I just heard from my oncologist that the MRI found brain mets. Most are located in the cerebellum (specifically the area that controls balance) and the frontal cortex. I am very frightened, not only because cancer has raised the stakes but also because my brain has been such a vehicle for enjoyment for me. I love to think and am dreading a future where irradiated holes in my brain make this less likely.

Because the news came after the medical offices were all closed, we have not been able to take any action. However, the plan is to get me an appointment with the fabulous radiation oncologist, who came to us from Johns Hopkins last year. We will see what she thinks and then the team will come to a decision as to next steps. Choices are either to wait and see if the chemo has an effect or to go ahead and irradiate one or more of these lesions.

Please hold me in your prayers. Cancer has just shoved this whole thing into hyperdrive and I can't help but think that my time is getting short. Once we have a plan I will let you know.

* * * *

Just a short update. My gamma knife surgery has been scheduled for Oct. 15. We will need to be in Spokane on the 14th when they will attach the halo to my head and do the mapping for the surgery. We are thinking that we might go to a nice lodge in Snoqualmie a few days prior to see the fall leaves and help pass the time. Meanwhile, the CT and bone scan I had recently confirm that my disease "below the neck" is behaving quite nicely as the chemo is doing its job. So I am relatively at ease over what is ahead. The palliative doc has been quite successful at finding a way around the fatigue and some of the gastrointestinal complaints so I am also much more comfortable. Now if I can lose the dizziness I think it will be manageable.

* * * *

It has been a week since I returned from Spokane and my grand adventure. We went a day early to play and had a good, albeit very gentle, time exploring downtown. The procedure went very smoothly and it was obvious that these guys know their stuff. Although I was at the clinic from 7am to 4:30pm the actual surgery only took three hours. They did find an extra, previously unknown, lesion and so were able to zap all three.

By far the most anxiety producing part was getting the frame, or halo, screwed into my skull. The local anesthetic hurt like h**l and they had to jab me in each of the four sites at least twice. The frame itself was titanium. (I was so tempted to sing "I am titanium!") So it was very light, which was good because I was wearing it from 8:00am until 4:00pm. After they bolted me to the table so I would be unable to move, they gave me conscious sedation. I don't remember anything except coming to in a big muddle as they were pulling me out of the machine.

As an example of how patient centered they are, they had recruited a nurse especially for me. She had had a trach for six months so knew how to clean one, all the things that could go wrong, and was there just in case something did. She was also very funny and there was much laughter surrounding me throughout the day. Another fun fact is that the week before they had switched out their old gamma knife machine for a brand new model with bells and whistles, one of which was that the machine was self-adjusting so they no longer had to stop everything to come in and reposition me for each of the three sites. I don't remember what they named their old machine but the new one was named Sven! Any practice that names its machines has got my respect and interest!

I was fortunate in not having to go back to the hospital for the night. We got back to the hotel and I hit the bed and didn't wake up for 14 hours. Bill drove us home and the scenery was breathtaking, as always. There are no ugly drives in Montana but that coupled with the aspens' gold and the larches' mustard blazing all along the route was glorious. We also were able to stop at Krispy Kreme in Spokane before we left and buy two dozen donuts to freeze and bring home. It was like a pilgrimage, it has been so long since I have had a decent donut!

For the next few days I had horrible headaches and nausea but finally they went away. The incision sites on my head are still swollen and sore and I look like I am glowering at the world but that will also go away in time. The next thing on the time line is that I will have an MRI here in Kalispell to see whether we achieved our goal, so just hanging out 'til then and getting chemo on my normal schedule.

Most of my doctors have said that the tumors were too small to have affected me (they looked much bigger to me when I finally saw the MRI) but whether it is the placebo effect or the surgery I am feeling better. The primary complaint now is my paralyzed stomach which really makes my life grim when it acts up. But, on days like yesterday when it is behaving, I feel absolutely wonderful! (Not behaving today.) Whereas before the surgery I felt my traveling days were numbered and I should hang up my skis, since the surgery I am feeling that I have a few more trips in me and might ski this season once I get into better condition.

Thank you all for your prayers. They made such a difference. Here is a story about the omen I was given that things would be OK: when I was being shown around the facility by my surgeon, Dr. McKay, on the day before, one of the nurses offered me bagpipe music during the procedure as a joke, and not knowing my Scottish interest. That led to us talking about Scotland and his stint training in Edinburgh and his daughter's field work excavating sites in Orkney. Then the physicist was standing nearby who had just been to Scotland to visit his family sites. The final "coincidence" is that McKay's daughter lives in Marion, Montana (just down the road about 25 miles) and he has just bought a condo in Kalispell near the hospital, which is most likely in our complex. So, good Scots with a love for Kalispell, I am being taken care of and this was a Godwink for sure!

* * * *

I got reports back today from both radiation oncology and cardiology on the tests last week. As with everything regarding advanced cancer the results were not clear and the way forward is murky. A friend calls cancer "Whack-a-mole" and that certainly is my experience because, as soon as you feel you can draw a deep breath and relax, something else comes at you and usually it is from an unexpected direction and completely pulls the rug out from under the stable footing you thought you had achieved.

My first report of the day was on the brain MRI. The nurse told me that it is too soon to tell how successful the surgery was; we will have a better idea at next follow-up in January. But two of the three lesions are looking like they may be on their way out. The third lesion still shows some signs of life but we won't know for awhile. Meanwhile, then she reminded me that the extreme levels of lethargy and fatigue are a result of the surgery, and that I can expect them to continue for a few months. This fatigue is the worst ever, and I am used to chemo related fatigue! Not only do you feel like you are moving while submerged in a vat of honey, you also feel like you have lactic acid build up in your muscles. Next, phone call consult with neurosurgeon from Spokane on Thursday.

So I was feeling pretty good after this and thought: "Yeah, I've got a few years yet." And then… I heard from my cardiologist. Wham! I was run over by a truck, hit from behind and flattened in the middle of the freeway.

To remind everyone, my cancer is HER2 positive. It is the most aggressive form of breast cancer, after inflammatory, but it has been corralled by the wonderful drug Herceptin which keeps the cancer growing slowly rather than exploding, which is what it would rather do if left to its own devices. It is all wonderful, except Herceptin can cause congestive heart failure, which I experienced a bit last year. Because we were able last year to reverse the cardiac failure I was able to go on a wonderful chemotherapy agent, Kadcyla, that puts the cytotoxin inside a molecule of Herceptin that then delivers the toxin to the cancer cell, thus sparing my normal cells and reducing side effects. However, because of last year's episode they are monitoring my heart closely.

The cardiologist told me that the most recent echo indicated that my heart is enlarging and that it is not pumping as strongly as it had been. I am to have another echo in December to see if this trend is continuing. Meanwhile, I have a call into my medical onc to see what we want to do vis-à-vis the chemotherapy regimen that I am on. Do we continue to use the Kadcyla and monitor the heart until it gets to some point of weakness? Do we change chemo agents right now and go on something that is not related to Herceptin that will spare my heart?

This will be a dance we do for the rest of my life. I am not looking forward to being off the Herceptin and watching my cancer grow like wildfire but at some point the cancer may become secondary to my heart failure. I think this qualifies as being caught between the devil and the deep blue sea!

* * * *

I just saw my oncologist to get the results of my most recent CT scan. The scan before this showed some "ground-glass opacity" in my lung. This CT shows the same plus a little worsening. We don't know what it is. Based on the way my cancer has behaved in my lungs in the past my oncologist does not believe that it is cancer. Plus, if it is cancer there isn't anything we can do that is different anyway. I have no fever and I am not coughing up blood which is good and I am feeling really well so I will just keep on and live with the uncertainty. Cancer is definitely teaching me how to do this! I am scheduled for next chest CT in 90 days and I will have a brain MRI around that time as well. Onward…

* * * *

My visit with my oncologist yesterday was good but once again opened up a bit of fear over this lung infection. I have had an area show up on my last two CT scans that looked like ground glass. As I had no symptoms the first time, we assumed that it would go away. Three months later the next scan showed it still there and it has grown in size. My oncologist does not believe that it is cancer by the look of it, although it could be a different type of cancer. If it is cancer my oncologist jokingly said that she didn't want to know as there are no more breast cancer treatment options available for me. If it is another type of cancer it will mean being on an additional chemotherapy which my body may not be able to stand.

Saw the scans and it is a pretty large area involved. Not sure I would be eligible for another lobectomy as I have already had one lobe taken out as well as multiple wedges of remaining lungs. Big likelihood I will have to have another lung biopsy in any event. It could be sarcoidosis, antibiotic resistant TB, or some form of pneumonia, even though I have had the Pneumovax. Symptoms still are light breathlessness (93 on pulse-ox without supplemental oxygen so pretty decent) and an increasing back pain. Three weeks until I see the pulmonologist. So meanwhile, I will make accommodation for the pain and continue to live my life. For me it will always be something!

I do want to get a POLST form signed by the doc and in the house just in case this all blows up. Just to refresh everyone's memory, you can have your advanced directive signed but it is a suggestion not a doctor's order. A POLST form is signed by a doctor, kept on your refrigerator door where the EMTs can find it, and it covers whether you are to be moved to the hospital, and what level of care you are to receive (i.e. including a DNR). This way if an ambulance comes to get you their actions will be prescribed by a physician which will override state laws on requiring artificial resuscitation.

Don't anticipate any other news until after the pulmonologist visit. Will update again after we know something. Meanwhile, spring is a good four weeks early this year and it is glorious! It is hard to feel badly when the view is so stupendous.

* * * *

I have good news! That doesn't happen often so I have to enjoy it when I can. After a month-long wait to get in to see the pulmonologist I finally saw him yesterday. I liked him tremendously. He has a brisk no-nonsense delivery that belies what I see and I have been told he has a very kind heart. He had read all of my file notes (which in itself is a noteworthy accomplishment being how extremely large and convoluted my history is), and after asking me a few questions about my history and my trach he sent me on a little walk around the office for six minutes tied to a pulse-ox monitor. Although I felt a bit winded my oxygen levels remained above 90% throughout.

He showed me my CT and explained that he thinks this is related to the radiation I received 11 years ago. While radiation-induced pulmonary fibrosis usually occurs within a few months to a couple of years following radiation, it has been known to appear years after the event.

He seconds my oncologist that this does not look like cancer. What is his major clue is that the ground-glass looking area is in the top and middle lobes of the right lung and is bounded by a straight line. Now, nothing in nature is a straight line (especially cancer) so this leads him to think that it has to do with the masking done during the original radiation. As to why now, well the best guess he can come up with is that the new chemo (which is much more powerful than any others taken here-to-date) has sensitized the tissue paving the way for this.

There is no cure for this and it will continue to get worse in all likelihood but should not affect my breathing as I am coping quite well right now. I get CT scans every three months anyway and I will just make sure he is copied on the list of docs who get copies and we will keep an eye out. If anything changes we should be able to catch it with this schedule.

I have begun to work out with BV's Parkinson's exercise group twice a week and can tell a difference in my general endurance as well as balance. My goal is a gentle hike in Glacier from the top of the Going-to-the-Sun Road toward the end of the summer. So thanks for the prayers. It is as good as the news could be and I thank your efforts for keeping me calm and positive while waiting. My next CT is next month and then my head MRI is scheduled in early Sept. so I will check in with you once I have news from those.

* * * *

The Kadcyla has stopped working. We met with my oncologist today and went over my, now very limited, options. All the drugs now are chemotherapy and highly toxic. We are having to choose between the side effects of neurotoxicity or heart toxicity so are opting for neurotoxicity at this point as my oncologist thinks this drug has the best chance of being effective. I do not qualify for many of the new therapies that are out there or for any clinical trials.

We have tentatively scheduled my first dose of the new medication for Sept. 23 and we will see how I do. I will update when we know more. This wrinkle has shown us that it is imperative to get nursing home options squared away so when I die Bill is cared for, but honestly I haven't got the energy. Maybe since I did not get treatment today I will have a burst of energy between now and then and can take care of this.

* * * *

I am feeling like there is something just not right so I called the folks at radiation oncology and asked if we could move up the brain MRI six weeks. As I have the reputation for feeling what's wrong long before I should be able to, they moved it right up. Just got the call back and the cancer has, in fact, returned to my brain. I do not know how many lesions nor do I know how large or where. I will see the radiation oncologist on Monday afternoon for full report and decision time.

I have a call into my medical oncologist to tell her what they found so she can have some time to think about whether that will change the chemo I am on. I was to see her on Wednesday morning but she may opt to move that appointment up as well as schedule the chest CT for now so we can get a complete picture.

It is hard to have hope when this happens, but it is also hard to have hope when you generally feel like shit. I guess it is impossible to parse through any of this until Monday. Just so very very sad right now.

On a more mundane note, Bill and I are having real difficulty cooking now. A friend has set up a Meal Train for me for people to volunteer to bring meals twice a week. We are also going to be meeting with a home helping agency to discuss the possibility of hiring a cook one day a week to prepare meals and fill up the freezer so we have access to good, nutritional, and reheatable food.

* * * *

I promised to let you know how things have developed. I am having the gamma knife procedure on my brain on Tuesday and look forward to having those spots gone. Since I last updated this site I have had a chest CT to see if my cancer is growing in my body. It is. The tumors in my chest and on my adrenal gland have all become significantly larger. The chemo I have been on is not working. I met with my oncologist and we have mapped out the new treatment plan which will switch me to a new agent called eribulin. However, before I can begin the infusions we have to make sure that my heart is strong enough so my oncologist and cardiologist are looking into this. If my heart cannot sustain the treatment I will go on carboplatin, a very old line drug.

I probably will have to have these gamma knife treatments on a regular basis. I have come to terms with this and it now is just part of the fabric of living with this disease. I cannot worry about running out of treatment options any longer. It will happen when it happens and fretting will not change anything. Living each day is becoming more difficult as the cumulative effect of nearly eight years of nonstop treatment is taking its toll. We are fortunate to be able to find help when we need it so we can stay in our home. So life continues. We will see how things go after this next week.

* * * *

There is a phrase in palliative and hospice care, "turning the corner." It refers to that moment when the body starts the active dying process. While I am not at that stage right now I am at the stage where my spirit has turned the corner. We are no longer playing with the conceit that I have much time left. I have decided to share the experience of dying with anyone who wants to know more.

* * * *

For those of you still on this journey with me, thank you. We are coming up to the difficult times shortly and I need your prayers more than ever. I am currently on the next to last chemo drug that is available to me. We will not know whether it is working for another 45 days. If it is working then, hallelujah, I can squeeze out a little more time. If it is not working then I will be forced onto the last drug available to me. Assuming I can tolerate that drug I will then have another 90 days to see how it is working. If it is working then I will ride it out as long as possible. However, once it stops working I will be forced to go on hospice and will most likely die within six months. No matter how prepared and clear-eyed I seem about this it still is like getting punched in the gut. To know I am leaving Bill is hideous; the despair on his face is unbearable to me.

I do not know what to pray for: another drug to come off the FDA approval line for yet more time, a change in hospice reimbursement so it will pay for Herceptin and gamma knife, for the drug I am on now to be effective until its replacement is available...

Please pray for the best outcome for my unfolding path, whatever that may be. And pray for Bill, that he receives the support he needs during this very confusing and unsettling time. And please pray for comfort when the tsunami of grief overwhelms us, like right now. As I figure it, worst-case scenario on average we would be looking at my dying in late September to early October.

* * * *

My follow-up chest scans have shown progression of the cancer. Based on this news I was expecting to be taken off the eribulin and be given the choice between going onto the last remaining chemo agent (Gemzar) or stopping treatment now and going into hospice. This is the way we have handled progression in the past and, based on the assumption that this time would be no different, I had been wrestling with my decision ever since I read the radiologist's report prior to my appointment with my oncologist.

My oncologist and I are in agreement that my body is exhausted from all that has gone before and cannot mount much of a defense and we do not expect that any chemo at this point can either have much effect or sustain it for very long. My quality of life is bounded by pain, extreme fatigue, and a host of other issues due to previous treatment. I know that I am going to die anyway and sometime relatively soon so I am ready to be done. Hospice is what I would choose if it wasn't for my concerns over Bill and his needs due to his Parkinson's.

But the decision-making mechanism has changed and I was surprised that the oncologist said that she did not think the progression was enough to require a change in treatment plan. This close to the end you must conserve your options in order to buy time. I am fortunate in that I do not have much tumor burden, and what I have is not life threatening in and of itself, so we have time for the existing tumors to continue to grow without putting my life at risk, which gives me more time even if the chemo is only marginally effective.

So, because of the flexibility this gives me, I will stay on the eribulin and we will monitor how quickly the cancer is growing and spreading. When the tumor burden gets greater and moves into new and life-threatening sites, like my liver, that is the time we will switch to the Gemzar and then ride that pony for as long as possible. If at any time it gets to be too much for me we can pull the plug and start hospice, so I am glad that I have that alternative available. Each day I have been deciding whether the suffering has been worth that day of life. Usually I can find reasons why it is so but the ratio of good days to bad days has now shrunk to about 50/50 and during chemo weeks it is 70% bad and only 30% good.

This new arrangement was not something that had even entered my mind, although it is extremely logical in hindsight. I have throughout this cancer experience had a number of times when I felt that my back was against the wall. At each of these times some light shines on the situation, even though I am without hope, and a new possibility opens up for me. It is enough to show me another, better, more hopeful way and to lead me through the valley. That these moments of grace appear right when they are so desperately needed is a testament to the continued prayer support of you and all those praying for me when I cannot find the words either due to fear or pain. So thank you again for accompanying me on this journey.

As for what is next, I have a follow-up MRI again of my brain in two weeks to check on how it is healing after the second gamma knife procedure last fall. I will have my next chest CT in three months unless something changes to demand it sooner. After that CT we will reevaluate next steps. Staying on the existing treatment (if nothing goes haywire) will add another three months to my life span which means that I may actually live to see Christmas again. I had not expected that so it is very exciting. Of course we don't know how I will react to the Gemzar but I am holding onto the hope that I can get three months out of it as well if not more.

I am not as greedy for life as I once was in this process, but I am full of curiosity as to how things will unfold and so the gentle joys of my days are more than satisfactory and I take them as a lovely gift and am thankful.

Part III: Turning the Corner

I will die soon. I don't know whether it will be in 6 months or 18, the factors are out of my control, but my spirit is making the adjustments that are needed for me to step between the worlds. I am noticing that the when of it is no longer important to me, which is an enormous surprise for someone who has fought for so long to beat the odds and stay around. It is a relief for me to be able to say these words 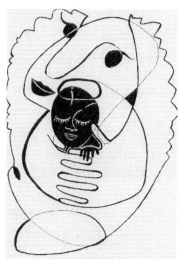 out loud and I am beyond grateful that my husband and I can talk about it as a fact, secure in the fact that our love for each other has been actualized every day of our married life and so we are OK.

A dear friend died two years ago and she was kind enough to e-mail me with notes from the frontier as she transitioned. It was a great gift that she gave me in describing her experience as being a gentle cocooning by loving spirits. I find this to be so as well.

I have done all I can with the things of this world that must be done: arrangements made, contracts signed, bequests made, preferences expressed. Now it is time for the soul work, the work that comes from a deep place out of sight and that can either be taken on or ignored. But I find that it isn't work and that, standing at somewhat a remove from this world now, it is just so very interesting to watch what is coming into my life to assist me.

When I was younger I began to notice a pattern during transitional periods in my life. Before I would be able to move along to the next thing, avatars for meaningful experiences and people of the time closing would suddenly appear in my life and offer an opportunity for me to address any unfinished business. The same thing is happening to me now.

My life has been characterized by hermetically sealed periods and identities. I was one of the people who experienced such family trauma as a child. The who I was was not acceptable to my parents and so it was ontologically critical that I develop a different way of being that would engage their care. This developed side of my personality became fiercely protective of the raw, soft, child that I was deep inside, but to the point of becoming dismissive of her in later life.

When I moved to Montana, it was to shed the fierce persona and to explore what I felt was my authentic, though neglected, self. I reconnected with friends from the old days but was surprised to realize that, in spite of myself, my entire personality had grown and changed. I was no longer the mountain girl who was comfortable living in a canyon and not seeing people for months on end, I needed engagement, I cared about the world, and I also needed a degree of creature comforts previously seen only as symbols of my other self.

The fact of living in a place of mountains and lakes and glaciers and fierce winds takes away the conceit of urban life that you have control. You don't have time to argue about turf when you are trying to survive a blizzard. You don't have time to thoroughly hate your neighbor if your survival is dependent upon your common life together. And so, in this clarifying environment, I was given a tremendous opportunity to see myself as I was and to learn that I was actually interesting and funny and worth knowing. It didn't matter that my in-laws never liked me, or that my mother never saw me, it didn't really make a dent or diminish me in any way that I didn't allow.

What is happening is that avatars of each stage of my life are appearing in my life now and will be part of my life at the end. The first thing that marked for me the new reality of approaching transition was a letter I received two years ago from the wife of my first love to tell me he had died suddenly of a heart attack. Although I was not in touch with him, this was a man to whom I had felt spiritually connected throughout my life. The idea of a world without his energy was unthinkable for me, he had been such a subliminal presence for over fifty years.

Two years ago through Facebook I was able to reconnect with a friend from my salad days when we were cool, fun, and rocking chicks. We were introduced at a family dinner and immediately clicked. And, at that time my fierce persona was tenaciously becoming French; my mother's Huguenot ancestry was a huge part of what Mother valued. It was an added benefit that this friend is French. Since those days we had lost touch. I am so glad to be back in touch with her.

The part of me that has been the most resistant to an inner-rapprochement has been the person I became when my fierce persona was allowed to run unchecked. I went into banking in my younger life because I knew that power followed money. Not having power made this decision a no-brainer for me, except that I am hopeless with numbers; I had a lot of work to do to try develop some facility with them. Ultimately this choice did lead to some really fun times once I had ascended the ladder, was running a corporate finance department, and playing with the big dogs.

What is painful to me now is looking back and seeing how easy it is to fall into the belief that you are entitled to your good fortune in some way. I did. I was pretty insufferable. A tangible sign of that is the memory of the day when I realized that I had paid more for a pair of shoes in my closet than six months' pay for the woman who faithfully took care of our house and us on a weekly basis. I had gone to value things more than people and almost lost my soul.

I had wanted to bury those memories, to pretend that I was never that person. As someone who engages the spiritual, this was never going to be an option for me. The spiritual life is not one where ducking and dodging bad behavior is the best strategy. So, right on schedule, I got two Facebook friend requests this past weekend from people that represent that time. It is with great interest that I watch what happens next as I relate to them and to the memories of how I was in those days. They are giving me a gift of their presence and an opportunity to heal this part of my past. I am extremely grateful.

Unless there is a miracle, my days are winding down. I find that I am gradually letting things go that previously might have been important. I am spending my time with friends and loved ones. I have rediscovered silliness and great guffaws of laughter. I hope to go to my death with twinkling eyes and a happy heart. I will miss this world and I will miss experiencing this world in the way that only a physical body can, but I will have absolutely no regrets.

Part IV: End Notes

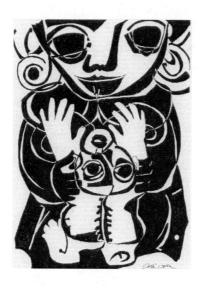

Glossary

Adjuvant therapy: treatment given following the initial diagnosis and surgery to lessen the odds that the cancer might recur.

Advanced directive: a document that expresses one's wishes as to life sustaining treatments that may be administered towards the end of life.

Alchemy: a process thought to turn base metals into gold.

Allopathic medicine: a medical system which uses drugs and other forms of treatment that have been proven to have benefit through clinical research.

Bell curve: a bell curve is a graphic image in the shape of a bell that expresses the expected normal distribution of cases of a variable. What is considered normal is whatever the majority represents. When plotted, this majority will fall graphically on the middle of the x-axis (representing the variable), and the number of cases (y-axis) will determine the depth of the dome of the bell, with fewer and fewer cases on either side the further the case is found from the center (the tails).

Biologic: a medicine that is used to bind to the surface of a tumor cell and to interfere with that cell's life sustaining and growth functions.

Biomedicine: a medical system that relies on knowledge of the biological sciences.

Chicken Little: a character from a children's story that exclaimed frequently that the sky was falling when it wasn't. Also known as Henny-Penny.

CT scan: computerized axial tomography. This is basically a high tech x-ray for viewing structures inside the body.

Cytotoxin: a medicine that poisons tumor cells.

Dame Julian: Julian of Norwich, a 14th century English Christian mystic.

DNR: a do not resuscitate order.

EMT: Emergency medical technician.

Hematocrit: the ratio of red blood cells to total blood cells. Too high or too low a figure could be a sign of a variety of illnesses, infection, or mineral and vitamin deficiencies.

HER2+: Human Epidermal Growth Factor Receptor 2 positive. A positive status indicates that the cancer is an aggressive, rapidly growing cancer. Fortunately, there are now drugs that successfully interfere with this process and can now slow the cancer's growth.

Metastatic Cancer: cancer that has spread outside of the original cancer site. In breast cancer the metastatic sites usually include: lungs, liver, bones, and brain. If the tumors that appear in these metastatic sites match the characteristics of the tumors in the primary site, or breast, the disease is still breast cancer and not brain cancer or bone cancer and is referred to as breast cancer with metastases to the brain, etc.

Metavivor: a person with Stage 4 metastatic breast cancer.

Monocytes: a type of white blood cell.

MRI: magnetic resonance imaging. This technology uses radio

waves to take pictures of structures inside the body.

Outlier: in medicine a case that does not meet the criteria that defines a normal or expected reaction to a medication or intervention. (See Bell curve above.)

PET scan: positron emission tomography uses a dye with radioactive material to see how the body is functioning.

POLST: a physician's order concerning life sustaining treatment. This order tells any emergency medical workers what sort of life sustaining measures, if any, are to be used.

Radiofrequency ablation: in cancer it is using electrical energy to burn out diseased tissue.

Ski-joring: a race over an obstacle course where a skier is pulled by an animal, usually a horse or a dog.

Thoracotomy: a surgery that involves opening the chest cavity to get access to the organs inside such as lungs and heart.

Titration: increasing or decreasing the dosage of medicines in steps over a period of time. Some medicines require this to enable the body to adjust to the desired therapeutic dose.

References

Brady, M.J.; Peterman, A.H.; Fitchett, G.; Mo, M.; Cella, D. (1999) "A case for including spirituality in quality of life measurement in oncology." *Psycho-Oncology*, 8, 417–428

Clark, D. (2000, July/August) "Total pain: The work of Cicely Saunders and the hospice movement." *APS Bulletin*, 10(4). Retrieved May 20, 2006, from American Pain Society Web site: http://www.ampainsoc.org/pub/bulletin/ju00/hist1.htm

Duff, K. (1993) *The Alchemy of Illness*. New York: Bell Tower

Goldstein, M.A. (2000) *Travels with the Wolf: A Story of Chronic Illness*. Columbus, Ohio: Ohio State University Press

Hunt, L.M. (2000) "Strategic Suffering: Illness Narratives as Social Empowerment among Mexican Cancer Patients." In C. Mattingly and L.C. Garro (Eds.), *Narrative and the Cultural Construction of Illness and Healing* (pp. 88–107). Berkeley: University of California Press

Kleinman, A. (1988) *The Illness Narratives: Suffering, Healing & the Human Condition*. New York: Basic Books

McGrath, P. (2002) "Creating a language for 'spiritual pain' through research: a beginning." *Supportive Care in Cancer*, 10, 637–646

Vance, L.M.F. (2007) *Spiritual Experiences of Chronic Illness when There is No Personal God*. Ann Arbor, Michigan: ProQuest

Young-Mason, J. (1997) *The Patient's Voice: Experiences of Illness*. Philadelphia: F.A. Davis Company

About the Author: Landis M.F. Vance

Landis Vance has been interested in the relationship between spiritual and physical health for many years. Feeling called to advocate for and bolster the spiritual growth that can come for those wrestling with the chaos of illness, she left a career to go back to graduate school to study the interrelationship between spirituality, religion, psychology, and medicine, receiving an interdisciplinary PhD in Practical Theology and Health from the Union Institute and University. She also was involved in field training as a hospital chaplain.

Since that time Dr. Vance has functioned as a chaplain in critical care and palliative care departments within research hospitals and urban trauma centers. She has also taught medical students the impact of culture, religion, and spirituality on therapeutic relationships and functioned as a mentor for both medical students and seminarians in formation and training.

Dr. Vance believes in knowledge that informs practice to make the ways we care for and are cared for more effective when in the chaos of illness, and particularly in the ongoing stress and loss of living with chronic illness. She also believes strongly that the trauma of illness is a spiritual trauma but that it can provide an opening for positive life changes and deepening spirituality if one is willing to confront its darkness and to hold tight for its blessing. While she continues to monitor the academic press in her field, her own knowledge has become more complex and nuanced as she, herself, is now living with a terminal cancer.

About the Artist: Csaba Osvath

Csaba Osvath is an artist of great empathy and power as well as a Christian pastor. He has studied and implemented various art media in the community and touched lives through his artistic interpretation in Hungary, Wales, and the United States. He has presented and exhibited in over 46 lectures and workshops on art and theology and taught, designed, and participated in solo and group art exhibitions nationwide.

Among his many degrees in theology and in the creative arts, he received a Doctor of Art and Theology degree from Wesley Theological Seminary. Dr. Osvath served the Hungarian Reformed Church in Washington, D.C., and he continues to serve in Sarasota, Florida. He also served as artist-in-residence at Arlington United Methodist Church and has dedicated his life to the prophetic voice through the visual arts, specializing in oil painting, pen and ink, mixed media, artistic performance, and sculpting.

The artworks provided in this book were created when Dr. Osvath and Dr. Vance worked together in the palliative care department of a major research hospital and are the means by which Dr. Osvath communicates the spiritual suffering and struggle of patients that he witnessed while doing his field work internship.

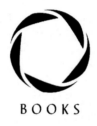

BOOKS

O-BOOKS

SPIRITUALITY

O is a symbol of the world, of oneness and unity; this eye represents knowledge and insight. We publish titles on general spirituality and living a spiritual life. We aim to inform and help you on your own journey in this life.
If you have enjoyed this book, why not tell other readers by posting a review on your preferred book site? Recent bestsellers from O-Books are:

Heart of Tantric Sex
Diana Richardson
Revealing Eastern secrets of deep love and intimacy to Western couples.
Paperback: 978-1-90381-637-0 ebook: 978-1-84694-637-0

Crystal Prescriptions
The A-Z guide to over 1,200 symptoms and their healing crystals
Judy Hall
The first in the popular series of four books, this handy little guide is packed as tight as a pill-bottle with crystal remedies for ailments.
Paperback: 978-1-90504-740-6 ebook: 978-1-84694-629-5

Take Me To Truth
Undoing the Ego
Nouk Sanchez, Tomas Vieira
The best-selling step-by-step book on shedding the Ego, using the teachings of *A Course In Miracles*.
Paperback: 978-1-84694-050-7 ebook: 978-1-84694-654-7

The 7 Myths about Love...Actually!
The journey from your HEAD to the HEART of your SOUL
Mike George
Smashes all the myths about LOVE.
Paperback: 978-1-84694-288-4 ebook: 978-1-84694-682-0

The Holy Spirit's Interpretation of the New Testament
A course in Understanding and Acceptance
Regina Dawn Akers
Following on from the strength of *A Course In Miracles*, NTI teaches us how to experience the love and oneness of God.
Paperback: 978-1-84694-085-9 ebook: 978-1-78099-083-5

The Message of A Course In Miracles
A translation of the text in plain language
Elizabeth A. Cronkhite
A translation of *A Course in Miracles* into plain, everyday language for anyone seeking inner peace. The companion volume, *Practicing a Course In Miracles*, offers practical lessons and mentoring.
Paperback: 978-1-84694-319-5 ebook: 978-1-84694-642-4

Rising in Love
My Wild and Crazy Ride to Here and Now, with Amma, the Hugging Saint
Ram Das Batchelder
Rising in Love conveys an author's extraordinary journey of

spiritual awakening with the Guru, Amma.
Paperback: 978-1-78279-687-9 ebook: 978-1-78279-686-2

Thinker's Guide to God
Peter Vardy
An introduction to key issues in the philosophy of religion.
Paperback: 978-1-90381-622-6

Your Simple Path
Find happiness in every step
Ian Tucker
A guide to helping us reconnect with what is really important in
our lives.
Paperback: 978-1-78279-349-6 ebook: 978-1-78279-348-9

365 Days of Wisdom
Daily Messages To Inspire You Through The Year
Dadi Janki
Daily messages which cool the mind, warm the heart and guide
you along your journey.
Paperback: 978-1-84694-863-3 ebook: 978-1-84694-864-0

Body of Wisdom
Women's Spiritual Power and How it Serves
Hilary Hart
Bringing together the dreams and experiences of women across
the world with today's most visionary spiritual teachers.
Paperback: 978-1-78099-696-7 ebook: 978-1-78099-695-0

Dying to Be Free
From Enforced Secrecy to Near Death to True Transformation
Hannah Robinson
After an unexpected accident and near-death experience,
Hannah Robinson found herself radically transforming her life,

while a remarkable new insight altered her relationship with her father; a practising Catholic priest.
Paperback: 978-1-78535-254-6 ebook: 978-1-78535-255-3

The Ecology of the Soul
A Manual of Peace, Power and Personal Growth for Real People in the Real World
Aidan Walker
Balance your own inner Ecology of the Soul to regain your natural state of peace, power and wellbeing.
Paperback: 978-1-78279-850-7 ebook: 978-1-78279-849-1

Not I, Not other than I
The Life and Teachings of Russel Williams
Steve Taylor, Russel Williams
The miraculous life and inspiring teachings of one of the World's greatest living Sages.
Paperback: 978-1-78279-729-6 ebook: 978-1-78279-728-9

On the Other Side of Love
A Woman's Unconventional Journey Towards Wisdom
Muriel Maufroy
When life has lost all meaning, what do you do?
Paperback: 978-1-78535-281-2 ebook: 978-1-78535-282-9

Practicing A Course In Miracles
A Translation of the Workbook in Plain Language and With Mentoring Notes
Elizabeth A. Cronkhite
The practical second and third volumes of The Plain-Language *A Course in Miracles*.
Paperback: 978-1-84694-403-1 ebook: 978-1-78099-072-9

Readers of ebooks can buy or view any of these bestsellers by clicking on the live link in the title. Most titles are published in paperback and as an ebook. Paperbacks are available in traditional bookshops. Both print and ebook formats are available online.

Find more titles and sign up to our readers' newsletter at http://www.johnhuntpublishing.com/mind-body-spirit

Follow us on Facebook at
https://www.facebook.com/OBooks/
and Twitter at https://twitter.com/obooks